Deliciously Diabetic: A Nourishing Renal Diet Cookbook for Healthy Kidneys

Savor Flavorful Meals While Nurturing Your Kidneys and Managing Diabetes

Dr. Charmain Wilson

Abstract

"Deliciously Diabetic: A Nourishing Renal Diet Cookbook for Healthy Kidneys" offers a carefully curated collection of delectable recipes tailored to meet the dietary needs of individuals managing both diabetes and kidney health.

This comprehensive cookbook presents a range of flavorful dishes, thoughtfully designed to maintain blood sugar levels and support renal function.

With a focus on nutrient-rich ingredients and mindful portioning, each recipe strikes a perfect balance between taste and health.

The cookbook provides essential guidance on ingredient substitutions, portion control, and nutritional information to empower readers in making informed food choices.

Whether newly diagnosed or seeking to enhance their well-being, this cookbook is an indispensable companion on the journey to better health and culinary delight.

Table of Contents

Introduction

In the realm of health and well-being, two prevalent conditions often intersect, demanding careful attention and specialised dietary considerations: diabetes and kidney disease. Both conditions require individuals to be vigilant about their food choices, making it essential to strike a delicate balance between managing blood sugar levels and supporting renal health. Recognizing this vital need, we proudly present "Deliciously Diabetic: A Nourishing Renal Diet Cookbook for Healthy Kidneys" – a comprehensive culinary guide meticulously crafted to empower individuals facing the dual challenge of diabetes and renal issues.

Managing diabetes and kidney disease simultaneously poses unique challenges, often requiring dietary restrictions and lifestyle adjustments. As the prevalence of these conditions continues to rise, individuals and their caregivers are seeking effective strategies to maintain quality of life while navigating the complex world of nutrition.

Emphasising the importance of maintaining a well-rounded, flavorful, and wholesome diet, this cookbook aims to inspire culinary creativity that not only satisfies the taste buds but also nurtures overall health.

At the core of this cookbook lies an array of thoughtfully curated recipes that artfully combine wholesome ingredients and innovative culinary techniques. With a focus on nutrient-rich foods, balanced macronutrients, and appropriate portion sizes, the recipes offer a harmonious fusion of flavors while ensuring glycemic control and promoting kidney well-being. We have taken care to meticulously develop each recipe, adhering to the dietary guidelines recommended for individuals with diabetes and kidney disease.

The journey to better health begins with knowledge and understanding. In the initial chapters, this cookbook delves into the fundamental principles of a diabetic renal diet, empowering readers with practical insights and guidelines. Readers will gain a comprehensive understanding of the interplay between blood sugar regulation and kidney function, along with tips on portion control, monitoring carbohydrate intake, and managing sodium and potassium levels.

One of the unique aspects of this cookbook is the versatility of its recipes, suitable for various dietary preferences and cultural backgrounds. Whether you are a vegetarian, vegan, or a fan of diverse global cuisines, "Deliciously Diabetic" caters to your individual taste and dietary requirements. Each recipe is accompanied by detailed nutritional information, helping readers make informed choices that align with their specific health needs.

In addition to the tantalising recipes, this cookbook also provides practical guidance on adapting recipes to accommodate dietary restrictions or allergies. Ingredient substitutions, cooking techniques, and storage tips empower readers to make flexible adjustments without compromising on flavor or nutritional value.

"Deliciously Diabetic" is more than just a cookbook; it is a compassionate companion for those embarking on a journey to better health and well-being. It advocates the idea that managing diabetes and kidney disease need not equate to sacrificing delicious food. Instead, it encourages a harmonious relationship between mindful eating and pleasurable dining.

In conclusion, "Deliciously Diabetic: A Nourishing Renal Diet Cookbook for Healthy Kidneys" sets out to inspire, educate, and empower readers to embark on a culinary adventure that celebrates both health and flavor. With its abundance of delectable recipes and essential dietary guidance, this cookbook becomes an indispensable tool for individuals seeking to savor the joy of cooking while fostering their overall well-being. Embrace this cookbook as your trusted ally, and let it be the first step towards a healthier, happier, and more flavorful life.

Chapter One

Understanding Diabetes and Kidney Health

Diabetes and kidney health are closely intertwined, with diabetes being one of the leading causes of kidney disease. The prevalence of diabetes has been steadily rising, which has resulted in a significant increase in cases of diabetic kidney disease, also known as diabetic nephropathy.

This chapter explores the intricate relationship between diabetes and kidney health, shedding light on the mechanisms, risk factors, and strategies for prevention and management.

1. The Link between Diabetes and Kidney Disease

The link between diabetes and kidney disease is a significant and intricate relationship that underscores the importance of managing blood glucose levels for overall health. Diabetes, especially type 2 diabetes, is a leading cause of kidney disease, known as diabetic kidney disease or diabetic nephropathy. Prolonged exposure to high blood glucose levels can damage the blood vessels in the kidneys, impairing their ability to function effectively.

The kidneys play a crucial role in filtering waste and excess fluids from the blood, maintaining a delicate balance of electrolytes and fluids, and producing hormones that regulate blood pressure. When blood glucose levels remain elevated over time, the delicate structures within the kidneys, such as the glomeruli and tubules, are affected. This damage can lead to protein leakage into the urine, reduced kidney function, and eventually, chronic kidney disease.

Early detection and management of diabetic kidney disease are vital to slow its progression and prevent further complications. Maintaining stable blood glucose levels through lifestyle modifications, proper medication adherence, and regular health check-ups are key factors in preserving kidney health for individuals living with diabetes. By understanding the link between diabetes and kidney disease, healthcare professionals and individuals can work together to implement proactive strategies that promote both diabetes management and kidney health.

2. Understanding Diabetic Nephropathy

Understanding diabetic nephropathy, also known as diabetic kidney disease, is essential for individuals with diabetes and healthcare professionals alike. Diabetic nephropathy is a progressive condition characterised by kidney damage due to prolonged exposure to high blood glucose levels in diabetes.

The kidneys, responsible for filtering waste and excess fluids from the blood, are highly vascular organs susceptible to damage from the effects of hyperglycemia. Over time, the tiny blood vessels (glomeruli) and tubules within the kidneys become impaired, leading to protein leakage into the urine (microalbuminuria) and declining kidney function.

The progression of diabetic nephropathy occurs in stages, starting with mild proteinuria and progressing to significant protein leakage (macroalbuminuria) and reduced kidney function. Left untreated, diabetic nephropathy can lead to end-stage renal disease (ESRD), requiring dialysis or kidney transplantation for survival.

Early detection of diabetic nephropathy is crucial for timely intervention and slowing disease progression. Regular health check-ups, kidney function tests, and urine albumin-to-creatinine ratio (UACR) assessments aid in identifying kidney damage in its initial stages.

Managing diabetic nephropathy involves controlling blood glucose levels, blood pressure, and other associated risk factors. Healthcare providers may prescribe medications such as angiotensin-converting enzyme inhibitors (ACE inhibitors) or angiotensin receptor blockers (ARBs) to protect kidney function and reduce proteinuria.

Through awareness, early detection, and comprehensive management, individuals with diabetes can take proactive steps to preserve kidney health and mitigate the impact of diabetic nephropathy on their overall well-being.

3. Risk Factors for Diabetic Kidney Disease

Risk factors for diabetic kidney disease, also known as diabetic nephropathy, play a crucial role in determining an individual's susceptibility to kidney complications in the presence of diabetes.

While diabetes itself is the primary risk factor, several other factors can influence the development and progression of diabetic kidney disease.

- **Poor Blood Glucose Control:** Prolonged exposure to high blood glucose levels (hyperglycemia) is the hallmark feature of diabetes and a significant risk factor for kidney damage. Consistently elevated blood glucose levels can lead to damage to the delicate blood vessels in the kidneys, impairing their filtration function.

- **Hypertension (High Blood Pressure):** Individuals with diabetes and uncontrolled hypertension are at a higher risk of diabetic kidney disease. High blood pressure puts additional strain on the blood vessels in the kidneys, exacerbating kidney damage.
- **Duration of Diabetes:** The longer an individual has diabetes, the higher the risk of developing diabetic nephropathy. Early onset and prolonged duration of diabetes increase the likelihood of kidney complications.
- Genetics: Family history of diabetic kidney disease or a genetic predisposition to kidney problems can elevate the risk of kidney damage in individuals with diabetes.
- **Smoking:** Smoking is a modifiable risk factor that can accelerate the progression of diabetic kidney disease. Quitting

smoking can help reduce the risk of kidney complications.

- **Coexisting Conditions:** Other health conditions, such as high cholesterol, obesity, and cardiovascular disease, can contribute to kidney damage in individuals with diabetes.
- **Age:** The risk of developing diabetic kidney disease tends to increase with age, making regular kidney health monitoring even more critical for older individuals with diabetes.

Understanding and addressing these risk factors are essential for preventing or slowing the progression of diabetic kidney disease. Regular health check-ups, blood glucose and blood pressure control, lifestyle modifications, and adherence to prescribed treatments are key elements in managing these risk factors and preserving kidney health for individuals living with diabetes.

4. Mechanisms of Kidney Damage in Diabetes

The mechanisms of kidney damage in diabetes are complex and involve a cascade of interrelated processes that are triggered by prolonged exposure to high blood glucose levels.

Chronic hyperglycemia leads to the formation of advanced glycation end-products (AGEs), which play a central role in the pathogenesis of kidney damage.

- **Formation of Advanced Glycation End-Products (AGEs):** High blood glucose levels can react with proteins and lipids in the body, leading to the formation of AGEs. These compounds accumulate in the kidneys and other tissues, promoting inflammation and oxidative stress.
- **Oxidative Stress:** The presence of AGEs and elevated glucose levels induce oxidative stress, resulting in an imbalance between reactive oxygen species (ROS) and antioxidants. Increased ROS levels cause damage to the cells and tissues of the kidneys.
- **Inflammation:** AGEs and oxidative stress trigger an inflammatory response within the kidneys, attracting immune cells and causing further tissue damage.

- **Activation of the Renin-Angiotensin-Aldosterone System (RAAS):** In response to kidney damage, the RAAS pathway becomes overactive, leading to increased blood pressure and further damage to the blood vessels in the kidneys.
- **Glomerular Hypertrophy and Hyperfiltration:** Chronic hyperglycemia causes the glomeruli, the tiny blood vessels in the kidneys responsible for filtration, to enlarge (glomerular hypertrophy) and filter more blood (hyperfiltration). This increased workload contributes to glomerular damage over time.
- **Fibrosis:** Prolonged inflammation and tissue damage lead to the accumulation of scar tissue (fibrosis) in the kidneys, impairing their ability to function properly.

These mechanisms collectively contribute to diabetic kidney disease or diabetic nephropathy. Early detection and management of kidney damage in diabetes are crucial for slowing disease progression and preserving kidney function.

Controlling blood glucose levels, blood pressure, and other associated risk factors can help mitigate the impact of these mechanisms on kidney health and overall well-being.

5. Diagnosing Diabetic Kidney Disease

Diagnosing diabetic kidney disease (DKD) is essential for early intervention and management to prevent further kidney damage. Regular kidney health monitoring is crucial for individuals with diabetes, as early detection can significantly impact disease progression and outcomes.

The primary diagnostic tools for DKD include:

I. Urine Albumin-to-Creatinine Ratio (UACR): This test measures the amount of albumin, a protein, in the urine relative to the amount of creatinine, a waste product. Elevated UACR levels indicate the presence of proteinuria, a hallmark sign of kidney damage.

II. Estimated Glomerular Filtration Rate (eGFR): The eGFR estimates how effectively the kidneys are filtering waste from the blood. A decline in eGFR indicates reduced kidney function.

III. Kidney Biopsy: In some cases, a kidney biopsy may be necessary to confirm the diagnosis and assess the severity of kidney damage. It entails taking a small sample of kidney tissue for microscopic examination.

Regular health check-ups and kidney function tests are essential for individuals with diabetes to monitor their kidney health. Early detection of kidney damage allows for timely intervention, including lifestyle modifications, blood glucose and blood pressure control, and medications such as angiotensin-converting enzyme inhibitors (ACE inhibitors) or angiotensin receptor blockers (ARBs) to protect kidney function.

Healthcare providers play a critical role in diagnosing and managing DKD, emphasizing the importance of routine screening and proactive measures to preserve kidney health for individuals living with diabetes.

6. Preventive Strategies for Diabetic Kidney Disease

Preventive strategies for diabetic kidney disease (DKD) are crucial in reducing the risk of kidney complications in individuals with diabetes. Early detection and intervention can significantly slow the progression of DKD and preserve kidney function.

Here are some preventive strategies:

I. Blood Glucose Control: Maintaining stable blood glucose levels through medication adherence, regular monitoring, and lifestyle modifications is fundamental in preventing DKD. Close collaboration with healthcare providers to set personalised blood glucose targets is essential.

II. Blood Pressure Management: Controlling hypertension is vital in preventing kidney damage. Lifestyle changes, such as a low-sodium diet, regular exercise, and stress reduction, along with prescribed medications, can help manage blood pressure effectively.

III. Healthy Diet: Adopting a balanced and kidney-friendly diet is beneficial in preventing DKD. Reducing salt, saturated fats, and processed foods and increasing the consumption of fruits, vegetables, and whole grains can support kidney health.

IV. Regular Exercise: Engaging in regular physical activity can help manage blood glucose levels, blood pressure, and body weight, all of which contribute to kidney health.

V. Avoiding Smoking and Limiting Alcohol: Smoking can accelerate kidney damage, and excessive alcohol consumption may strain the kidneys. Quitting smoking and moderating alcohol intake can support overall kidney health.

VI. Regular Kidney Function Tests: Routine monitoring of kidney function through tests like urine albumin-to-creatinine ratio (UACR) and estimated glomerular filtration rate (eGFR) helps in early detection of DKD.

VII. Medication Adherence: Taking prescribed medications, such as ACE inhibitors or ARBs, as directed by healthcare providers can help protect kidney function.

By implementing these preventive strategies and maintaining a proactive approach to diabetes management, individuals can significantly reduce the risk of diabetic kidney disease and maintain optimal kidney health. Collaboration with healthcare professionals in developing personalized prevention plans is essential for successful outcomes.

7. Lifestyle Modifications for Diabetes and Kidney Health

Lifestyle modifications play a pivotal role in managing both diabetes and kidney health. By adopting positive lifestyle changes, individuals can enhance their overall well-being and reduce the risk of complications associated with these conditions.

I. Balanced Diet: A well-rounded diet is essential for diabetes and kidney health. Pay attention to whole foods, such as fresh produce, whole grains, lean meats, and healthy fats. Limiting processed foods, added sugars, and excessive salt can benefit both conditions.

II. Carbohydrate Management: For individuals with diabetes, monitoring carbohydrate intake is crucial for blood glucose control. Opt for complex carbohydrates with a lower glycemic index, such as whole grains and legumes, to prevent spikes in blood sugar levels.

III. Blood Pressure Control: Managing blood pressure is vital for kidney health. Adopting a low-sodium diet, engaging in regular physical activity, and taking prescribed medications can help control hypertension.

IV. Regular Exercise: Physical activity is beneficial for both diabetes and kidney health. Regular exercise can improve blood glucose control, blood pressure, and cardiovascular health, supporting overall well-being.

V. Hydration: Maintaining a healthy level of hydration is crucial for kidney function. Aim to drink an adequate amount of water daily, unless advised otherwise by a healthcare provider due to specific medical conditions.

VI. Smoking Cessation: Smoking can exacerbate kidney damage and worsen diabetes-related complications. Quitting smoking can improve overall health and reduce the risk of kidney disease progression.

VII. Stress Management: Chronic stress can impact blood glucose levels and blood pressure. Adopt stress-reducing practices such as mindfulness, meditation, or yoga to promote well-being.

By incorporating these lifestyle modifications into their daily routines, individuals can optimise their diabetes management, protect kidney health, and reduce the risk of complications. Regular communication with healthcare providers is essential to develop personalised lifestyle plans and ensure the best possible outcomes for diabetes and kidney health.

8. Medications and Therapies for Diabetic Kidney Disease

Medications and therapies play a crucial role in managing diabetic kidney disease (DKD) and slowing its progression. Healthcare providers prescribe specific medications to protect kidney function, manage blood pressure, and reduce proteinuria.

Here are some common medications and therapies for DKD:

I. Angiotensin-Converting Enzyme Inhibitors (ACE Inhibitors) and Angiotensin Receptor Blockers (ARBs): These medications are the cornerstone of DKD management. They work by dilating blood vessels, reducing blood pressure, and protecting the kidneys from the damaging effects of high blood pressure. ACE inhibitors and ARBs also reduce proteinuria, which helps preserve kidney function.

II. Diuretics: Diuretics help control fluid retention and reduce edema (swelling) caused by kidney dysfunction. They can be prescribed to manage high blood pressure and fluid overload.

III. Sodium-Glucose Cotransporter-2 (SGLT2) Inhibitors: SGLT2 inhibitors are a class of medications that lower blood glucose levels by promoting glucose excretion in the urine. Recent studies have shown that SGLT2 inhibitors also provide renal benefits, including slowing the progression of DKD and reducing the risk of kidney failure.

IV. Statins: Statins are cholesterol-lowering medications that may be prescribed to manage high cholesterol levels in individuals with DKD. They can help reduce the risk of cardiovascular complications and may have additional benefits for kidney health.

V. Erythropoiesis-Stimulating Agents (ESAs): In cases where DKD has led to anaemia (low red blood cell count), ESAs may be prescribed to stimulate red blood cell production.

VI. Kidney Replacement Therapy: In advanced stages of DKD, when kidney function is severely impaired, kidney replacement therapy options like dialysis or kidney transplantation may be necessary to sustain life.

The choice of medications and therapies depends on the individual's specific health needs and the stage of DKD. Regular monitoring by healthcare providers is essential to adjust treatment plans as needed and optimise kidney health outcomes for individuals with DKD.

9. Nutritional Considerations for Diabetes and Kidney Health

Nutritional considerations are of utmost importance for individuals managing both diabetes and kidney health. A balanced diet can help regulate blood glucose levels, support kidney function, and minimise the risk of complications.

Here are some key nutritional considerations for diabetes and kidney health:

I. Manage Carbohydrate Intake: For individuals with diabetes, monitoring carbohydrate intake is essential for controlling blood glucose levels. Choosing complex carbohydrates with a low glycemic index can help prevent sharp spikes in blood sugar.

II. Protein Moderation: While protein is essential for the body, excessive protein intake can strain the kidneys. Individuals with kidney disease may need to limit protein consumption and focus on high-quality protein sources such as lean poultry, fish, and plant-based proteins.

III. Monitor Sodium (Salt) Intake: Reducing sodium intake can help manage blood pressure and prevent fluid retention. Limiting processed and packaged foods, which are often high in sodium, is crucial for kidney health.

IV. Balance Potassium and Phosphorus: Individuals with kidney disease may need to monitor potassium and phosphorus intake, as impaired kidney function can lead to imbalances. Healthcare providers may provide guidance on foods to include or limit in the diet.

V. Keep Hydrated: Kidney health depends on maintaining adequate hydration. Drinking enough water helps the kidneys flush out waste and toxins from the body.

VI. Limit Added Sugars and Saturated Fats: Reducing added sugars and saturated fats can help manage blood glucose levels and support heart health, reducing the risk of cardiovascular complications often associated with diabetes and kidney disease.

Individualised meal plans, developed in collaboration with registered dietitians or healthcare providers, are essential for addressing the unique nutritional needs of individuals with diabetes and kidney disease. Regular monitoring of blood glucose levels and kidney function, along with lifestyle modifications, can help optimise nutritional choices and promote overall well-being for those managing both conditions.

10. Importance of Blood Glucose Control

The importance of blood glucose control cannot be overstated for individuals with diabetes. Maintaining stable blood glucose levels is a cornerstone of diabetes management and is vital for overall health and well-being.

Here are some key reasons why blood glucose control is crucial:

I. Preventing Complications: High blood glucose levels over time can lead to a wide range of complications, such as diabetic retinopathy (eye damage), diabetic neuropathy (nerve damage), and diabetic nephropathy (kidney damage). By controlling blood glucose levels, individuals can significantly reduce the risk of these complications.

II. Managing Symptoms: Uncontrolled blood glucose can cause symptoms such as frequent urination, excessive thirst, fatigue, and blurred vision. Achieving optimal blood glucose control can alleviate these symptoms and improve quality of life.

III. Promoting Heart Health: High blood glucose levels can damage blood vessels and increase the risk of cardiovascular diseases, including heart attacks and strokes. Proper blood glucose control helps support heart health and reduces the risk of these complications.

IV. Enhancing Energy Levels: Stable blood glucose levels provide a consistent source of energy for the body. Avoiding extreme fluctuations in blood glucose can help individuals feel more energetic and better able to engage in daily activities.

V. Supporting Kidney Health: Blood glucose control is essential for preventing diabetic kidney disease and preserving kidney function. Managing blood glucose levels can reduce the strain on the kidneys and protect them from damage.

Regular blood glucose monitoring, adherence to prescribed medications, a balanced diet, regular physical activity, and ongoing communication with healthcare providers are essential components of achieving and maintaining blood glucose control. With diligent management, individuals with diabetes can significantly improve their overall health and reduce the risk of long-term complications.

In Summary

Understanding the intricacies of diabetes and kidney health is crucial in managing these conditions effectively. Early detection, regular monitoring, lifestyle modifications, and adherence to prescribed treatments are essential components of a comprehensive approach to mitigating the impact of diabetes on kidney function.

By fostering awareness and adopting proactive measures, individuals can enhance their overall well-being and maintain optimal kidney health in the presence of diabetes.

Chapter Two

Navigating a Diabetic Renal Diet: A Comprehensive Guide

For individuals managing both diabetes and kidney health, a diabetic renal diet is a critical component of their overall treatment plan.

A diabetic renal diet aims to strike a delicate balance between controlling blood glucose levels and supporting kidney function while minimizing the risk of complications associated with diabetic kidney disease (DKD).

This comprehensive guide explores all aspects of navigating a diabetic renal diet, including understanding the diet's principles, creating personalised meal plans, adapting recipes, addressing special dietary needs, and optimising nutrient intake.

Section 1: Understanding the Diabetic Renal Diet

A. The Importance of a Diabetic Renal Diet

The importance of a diabetic renal diet cannot be overstated for individuals managing both diabetes and kidney health. A well-planned diabetic renal diet is designed to support kidney function while managing blood glucose levels, reducing the risk of diabetic kidney disease (DKD) and its complications.

1. Controlling Blood Glucose Levels: A diabetic renal diet focuses on managing carbohydrates, choosing low glycemic index foods, and promoting stable blood glucose levels. By controlling blood glucose, individuals can reduce the risk of diabetes-related complications and prevent further kidney damage.

2. Supporting Kidney Health: The kidneys play a crucial role in filtering waste and maintaining fluid and electrolyte balance. A diabetic renal diet reduces the workload on the kidneys by limiting protein and sodium intake and balancing potassium and phosphorus levels. This approach helps preserve kidney function and slows the progression of diabetic kidney disease.

3. Reducing Complications: Diabetic kidney disease can lead to serious complications such as cardiovascular disease and end-stage renal failure. A diabetic renal diet helps manage blood pressure, lower inflammation, and maintain overall health, reducing the risk of these complications.

4. Personalized Approach: Each individual's dietary needs and health status are unique. A diabetic renal diet is tailored to address specific health concerns, making it an effective and sustainable approach to managing both diabetes and kidney health.

By adhering to a diabetic renal diet and collaborating with healthcare providers, individuals can take control of their health, improve quality of life, and reduce the impact of diabetes on kidney function.

1. Managing Carbohydrates

Controlling carbohydrates is a critical aspect of diabetes management, as it directly impacts blood glucose levels. For individuals with diabetes, understanding how different carbohydrates affect blood sugar and making appropriate dietary choices can help maintain stable glucose levels.

- **Choosing Complex Carbohydrates:** Complex carbohydrates, found in whole grains, legumes, and non-starchy vegetables, have a lower glycemic index compared to simple carbohydrates. They are digested more slowly, leading to a gradual rise in blood glucose levels, which is beneficial for diabetes management.
- **Monitoring Portion Sizes:** Keeping track of carbohydrate portions is essential for individuals with diabetes. Balancing carbohydrate intake with protein and healthy fats can prevent rapid spikes in blood sugar and help maintain more stable levels throughout the day.
- **Avoiding Sugary Foods:** Sugary foods and beverages, such as candies, pastries, and sugary

drinks, can cause sharp increases in blood glucose levels. Limiting or avoiding these high-sugar options supports better glucose control.

- **Timing of Carbohydrate Intake:** Spacing out carbohydrate consumption evenly throughout the day can help avoid large fluctuations in blood glucose levels. Eating balanced meals and snacks at regular intervals can promote better glucose management.

- **Blood Glucose Monitoring:** Regularly monitoring blood glucose levels allows individuals to assess how different foods and meals impact their blood sugar. This information helps make informed decisions about carbohydrate choices and meal planning.

- **Collaborating with Healthcare Providers:** Working closely with healthcare providers, such as registered dietitians and diabetes educators, can provide personalised guidance and meal planning strategies to manage carbohydrates effectively.

By managing carbohydrates wisely, individuals with diabetes can achieve better blood glucose control, reduce the risk of diabetes-related complications, and enhance their overall well-being. A balanced approach to carbohydrate intake is essential in diabetes management and supports a healthy lifestyle.

2. Limiting Protein Intake

Limiting protein intake is an essential aspect of a diabetic renal diet for individuals with kidney disease. While protein is a vital nutrient for the body, excessive protein consumption can strain the kidneys and worsen kidney function in individuals with impaired renal function.

• **Protecting Kidney Function:** The kidneys play a crucial role in filtering waste products and excess substances, including protein by-products. For individuals with kidney disease, reducing protein intake lessens the workload on the kidneys, helping to preserve their function and slow the progression of kidney damage.

• **Balancing Protein Quality:** Instead of restricting protein entirely, focusing on high-quality protein sources is recommended. Lean poultry, fish, and plant-based proteins such as legumes and tofu are preferred choices as they produce fewer waste by-products that must be filtered by the kidneys.

• **Managing Protein Portions:** Monitoring portion sizes of protein-rich foods is crucial to avoid excessive protein intake. Controlling protein portions while still meeting nutritional needs ensures a balanced diet that supports kidney health.

- **Collaborating with Healthcare Providers:** Working with registered dietitians or healthcare providers can help individuals determine their specific protein needs based on their stage of kidney disease and overall health. Personalised dietary recommendations ensure individuals receive adequate nutrients without overburdening the kidneys.

By carefully managing protein intake, individuals with kidney disease can protect their kidney function and support their overall health. Collaborating with healthcare providers and following a well-balanced diabetic renal diet contribute to better diabetes and kidney management, leading to improved quality of life.

3. Monitoring Sodium (Salt) Intake

Monitoring sodium intake is a crucial aspect of managing both diabetes and kidney health. Excessive sodium consumption can lead to increased blood pressure and fluid retention, placing added strain on the kidneys and potentially exacerbating kidney disease.

- **Blood Pressure Control:** High sodium intake is associated with elevated blood pressure, a significant risk factor for kidney disease and cardiovascular complications. Reducing sodium intake helps manage blood pressure, promoting kidney health and overall cardiovascular well-being.
- **Fluid Balance:** The body's fluid balance is significantly influenced by sodium. Excessive sodium can cause fluid retention, which can be particularly problematic for individuals with compromised kidney function. Limiting sodium intake helps maintain a proper fluid balance and reduces the risk of edema and other fluid-related issues.
- **Kidney Function Support:** By limiting sodium intake, individuals can ease the workload on the kidneys, promoting kidney function and reducing the risk of further damage. Managing sodium intake is especially important for individuals with existing kidney disease.
- **Reading Labels and Making Informed Choices:** Monitoring sodium intake requires reading food labels and making conscious choices when selecting foods. Opting for fresh, whole foods and avoiding processed and packaged items that often contain

high levels of sodium is essential for maintaining a healthy diet.

- **Collaborating with Healthcare Providers:** Working with registered dietitians or healthcare providers can provide valuable guidance on appropriate sodium intake based on individual health needs and kidney function. Personalised recommendations ensure individuals strike the right balance in their sodium consumption.

By carefully monitoring sodium intake and making informed choices, individuals can support their kidney health, manage blood pressure, and reduce the risk of complications associated with diabetes and kidney disease. A well-balanced diabetic renal diet, combined with sodium awareness, contributes to overall well-being and improved management of both conditions.

4. Balancing Potassium and Phosphorus

Balancing potassium and phosphorus intake is crucial for individuals managing both diabetes and kidney health. The kidneys play a vital role in regulating these electrolytes, and individuals with kidney disease may experience imbalances that can impact overall health.

- **Potassium Balance:** Potassium is essential for nerve and muscle function, including the heart. However, in kidney disease, impaired kidney function can lead to high potassium levels (hyperkalemia), which can be dangerous. Limiting potassium intake helps prevent hyperkalemia and reduces the risk of heart arrhythmias and other complications.

- **Phosphorus Balance:** Phosphorus is essential for bone health and energy production. In kidney disease, the kidneys may struggle to remove excess phosphorus, leading to elevated levels (hyperphosphatemia). High phosphorus levels have been linked to cardiovascular problems and bone thinning. Managing phosphorus intake supports bone health and reduces the risk of complications.

- **Food Choices:** Balancing potassium and phosphorus requires being mindful of food choices. Some foods, such as bananas, oranges, and tomatoes, are high in potassium, while dairy products and certain processed foods are rich in phosphorus. Choosing lower-potassium and lower-phosphorus options can help maintain a proper balance.

- **Working with Healthcare Providers:** Collaboration with registered dietitians and healthcare providers is essential for managing potassium and phosphorus intake. These experts can provide personalized dietary recommendations based on individual kidney function and health needs.

By balancing potassium and phosphorus intake, individuals can support kidney health, prevent electrolyte imbalances, and reduce the risk of complications associated with diabetes and kidney disease. Making informed food choices and seeking professional guidance contribute to an effective diabetic renal diet and overall well-being.

5. Adequate Fluid Intake

Adequate fluid intake is a vital aspect of managing both diabetes and kidney health. Staying hydrated is essential for maintaining overall well-being and supporting proper kidney function.

- **Kidney Health:** The kidneys rely on adequate fluid intake to effectively filter waste and toxins from the blood, producing urine to eliminate these substances from the body. Staying hydrated helps the kidneys maintain their function, reducing the risk of kidney damage and kidney stones.

- **Blood Glucose Control:** Proper hydration supports stable blood glucose levels. Dehydration can lead to elevated blood sugar levels, as the kidneys may conserve fluid, resulting in higher glucose concentrations in the blood. Maintaining adequate fluid intake helps manage blood glucose and supports diabetes management.

- **Electrolyte Balance:** Sufficient fluid intake is crucial for maintaining electrolyte balance, including sodium, potassium, and calcium. Proper electrolyte balance is essential for nerve and muscle function and overall health.

- **Preventing Dehydration:** Dehydration can lead to a range of health issues, such as fatigue, dizziness, and constipation. For individuals with diabetes, dehydration can exacerbate diabetes-related complications and increase the risk of kidney problems.

- **Individual Needs:** Fluid needs vary based on factors such as age, activity level, climate, and health status. Collaborating with healthcare providers to determine appropriate fluid intake based on individual needs ensures optimal hydration.

By maintaining adequate fluid intake, individuals can support kidney health, manage blood glucose levels, and promote overall well-being. Staying hydrated is a simple yet powerful aspect of a well-balanced diabetic renal diet that contributes to effective diabetes and kidney management.

C. Creating a Diabetic Renal Meal Plan

1. Understanding Individual Nutritional Needs
Understanding individual nutritional needs is a fundamental aspect of managing both diabetes and kidney health effectively. Each person has unique dietary requirements based on various factors, including age, gender, activity level, underlying health conditions, and kidney function.

- **Personalized Meal Planning:** Tailoring meal plans to individual nutritional needs ensures that essential nutrients are provided while avoiding excessive intake of certain substances that may pose risks to health.
- **Diabetes Management:** For individuals with diabetes, understanding their carbohydrate tolerance,

insulin requirements, and blood glucose response to different foods is crucial in creating personalised meal plans that support stable blood sugar levels.

- **Kidney Function:** For individuals with kidney disease, understanding their kidney function helps determine appropriate protein, sodium, potassium, and phosphorus intake to support kidney health and prevent further damage.

- **Food Preferences and Allergies:** Personal food preferences and any dietary allergies or intolerances must be considered when planning meals. Creating enjoyable and satisfying meals that align with individual tastes enhances adherence to the dietary plan.

- **Lifestyle Factors:** An individual's lifestyle, including work schedule, physical activity level, and social commitments, can influence dietary choices and meal timings. Considering these factors helps create practical and sustainable dietary plans.

- **Collaboration with Healthcare Providers:** Working with registered dietitians and healthcare providers ensures a comprehensive assessment of individual nutritional needs and provides expert guidance on tailoring meal plans to support diabetes and kidney health effectively.

Understanding individual nutritional needs empowers individuals to make informed choices about their diet, leading to better diabetes and kidney management. A personalised approach to meal planning enhances adherence, promotes overall well-being, and supports a healthy lifestyle for individuals navigating the challenges of diabetes and kidney health.

2. Balancing Macronutrients

Balancing macronutrients is a key principle of a well-rounded diabetic renal diet that supports both diabetes management and kidney health.

Proper balance of carbohydrates, proteins, and fats ensures optimal nutrition and stable blood glucose levels.

- **Carbohydrates:** Monitoring carbohydrate intake is essential for individuals with diabetes as they significantly impact blood glucose levels. Choosing complex carbohydrates with a low glycemic index, such as whole grains, legumes, and non-starchy vegetables, helps regulate blood sugar and prevents spikes.
- **Proteins:** While protein is crucial for tissue repair and muscle function, limiting protein intake is

important for individuals with kidney disease to reduce the burden on the kidneys. Choosing lean protein sources like poultry, fish, and plant-based options, while moderating portions, supports kidney health.

- **Fats:** Healthy fats, such as those found in avocados, nuts, and olive oil, provide essential fatty acids and support heart health. Balancing fat intake helps manage cholesterol levels and promotes overall cardiovascular well-being.

- **Portion Control:** Monitoring portion sizes of macronutrients is vital for diabetes and kidney management. Proper portion control ensures a balanced intake of nutrients and helps maintain stable blood glucose levels.

- **Personalized Meal Planning:** Tailoring macronutrient ratios to individual needs and health goals ensures that the dietary plan aligns with diabetes and kidney management requirements, promoting optimal health outcomes.

By carefully balancing macronutrients, individuals can maintain stable blood glucose levels, support kidney function, and prevent diabetes-related complications. Collaborating with healthcare providers and registered dietitians is crucial in creating personalised meal plans that optimise nutrition, contributing to overall well-being and improved management of diabetes and kidney health.

3. Portion Control

Portion control is a critical component of managing both diabetes and kidney health. It involves understanding and managing the quantity of food consumed in each meal and snack, which plays a significant role in maintaining stable blood glucose levels and supporting kidney function.

- **Blood Glucose Management:** Controlling portion sizes helps individuals with diabetes manage their blood glucose levels effectively. Overeating can lead to spikes in blood sugar, while consuming insufficient carbohydrates may cause hypoglycemia. Proper portion control ensures a balanced intake of nutrients, promoting stable blood glucose levels throughout the day.
- **Kidney Function Support:** For individuals with kidney disease, portion control is essential to prevent excessive strain on the kidneys. Overconsumption of protein or certain minerals like sodium and phosphorus can exacerbate kidney

damage. Managing portion sizes helps ease the workload on the kidneys and slows the progression of kidney disease.

• **Weight Management:** Portion control contributes to weight management, which is crucial for individuals with diabetes and kidney health. Maintaining a healthy weight helps improve insulin sensitivity, reduce the risk of diabetes-related complications, and support overall well-being.

• **Mindful Eating:** Practising portion control encourages mindful eating, which involves savouring food, recognizing hunger and satiety cues, and being present during meals. Mindful eating fosters a healthy relationship with food and can help prevent overeating.

• **Collaboration with Healthcare Providers:** Healthcare providers and registered dietitians can offer guidance on appropriate portion sizes based on individual needs and health goals. Personalised portion control recommendations optimise nutrition and enhance diabetes and kidney management.

By practising portion control, individuals can maintain stable blood glucose levels, support kidney health, and promote overall well-being. Being mindful of portion sizes and seeking professional guidance ensures a well-balanced diabetic renal diet, contributing to effective management of diabetes and kidney health.

4. Regular Meal Times

Regular meal times are an essential aspect of managing both diabetes and kidney health. Consistent meal timings play a significant role in regulating blood glucose levels, supporting digestion, and maintaining overall well-being.

- **Blood Glucose Management:** Eating meals at regular intervals helps stabilize blood glucose levels. Consistent meal times facilitate better insulin utilization and glycemic control, reducing the risk of blood sugar fluctuations and diabetes-related complications.
- **Appetite Regulation:** Establishing regular meal times aids in regulating appetite and preventing excessive hunger. This can prevent overeating and promote healthier food choices, supporting weight management and diabetes control.
- **Digestive Health:** Following a routine meal schedule allows the digestive system to function optimally. Consistent meal times support proper

digestion and nutrient absorption, contributing to overall gastrointestinal health.

• **Medication Management:** For individuals with diabetes, regular meal times help synchronise meal planning with medication schedules. This ensures that medications, such as insulin or oral hypoglycemic agents, are taken at appropriate times to match the body's glucose needs.

• **Energy Levels:** Consistent meal times provide a steady supply of energy throughout the day. Maintaining energy levels supports productivity, physical activity, and mental alertness.

• **Collaboration with Healthcare Providers:** Healthcare providers and registered dietitians can offer personalised recommendations for meal timing based on individual needs and health goals. Adhering to a regular meal schedule optimises nutrition and enhances diabetes and kidney management.

By following regular meal times, individuals can regulate blood glucose levels, promote proper digestion, and support overall health. Establishing a routine meal schedule and collaborating with healthcare providers create a solid foundation for a well-balanced diabetic renal diet, contributing to effective diabetes and kidney management.

5. Nutrient-Rich Ingredients

Nutrient-rich ingredients are the foundation of a well-rounded diabetic renal diet that supports both diabetes management and kidney health. These ingredients are packed with essential vitamins, minerals, and antioxidants, providing numerous health benefits.

- **Fruits and Vegetables:** Fruits and vegetables are rich in vitamins, minerals, fiber, and antioxidants, which are essential for overall health. They promote digestive health, support immune function, and help manage blood glucose levels.
- **Whole Grains:** Whole grains, such as brown rice, quinoa, and oats, are excellent sources of complex carbohydrates and fiber. They help regulate blood glucose levels, promote satiety, and provide sustained energy.
- **Lean Proteins:** Lean protein sources, including poultry, fish, legumes, and tofu, offer high-quality protein without excessive saturated fat or phosphorus. Adequate protein intake supports tissue repair, muscle function, and overall health.

- **Healthy Fats:** Healthy fats, such as those found in avocados, nuts, and olive oil, provide essential fatty acids that support heart health and reduce inflammation.
- **Nuts and Seeds:** Nuts and seeds are nutrient powerhouses, offering a blend of protein, healthy fats, vitamins, and minerals. They contribute to heart health and support weight management.
- **Dairy Alternatives:** For individuals with kidney disease, dairy alternatives like almond or soy milk provide essential nutrients without high phosphorus content.
- **Herbs and Spices:** Herbs and spices add flavour and aroma to dishes without added sodium. They possess various health-promoting properties, including anti-inflammatory and antioxidant effects.

Incorporating nutrient-rich ingredients into the diet helps optimise nutrition, promote overall well-being, and support diabetes and kidney management. A varied and balanced selection of these ingredients forms the basis of a diabetic renal diet that contributes to enhanced health outcomes and improved quality of life.

1. Lowering Sodium

Lowering sodium intake is a crucial dietary strategy for managing both diabetes and kidney health. Excessive sodium consumption can lead to elevated blood pressure, fluid retention, and increased strain on the kidneys, posing significant risks to cardiovascular and renal health.

• **Blood Pressure Control:** High sodium intake is associated with hypertension, a significant risk factor for heart disease and kidney damage. Reducing sodium helps maintain healthy blood pressure levels, promoting overall cardiovascular well-being.

• **Kidney Function Support:** The kidneys play a vital role in regulating sodium levels in the body. Lowering sodium intake reduces the workload on the kidneys, supporting their function and slowing the progression of kidney disease.

• **Fluid Balance:** Excess sodium can lead to fluid retention, causing edema and exacerbating heart and kidney conditions. Reducing sodium intake helps maintain a proper fluid balance in the body.

- **Reading Food Labels:** Monitoring sodium intake requires reading food labels to identify hidden sources of sodium in processed and packaged foods. Choosing low-sodium alternatives supports a healthier diet.

- **Cooking and Meal Preparation:** Limiting added salt during cooking and meal preparation helps lower sodium content in meals. Instead, using herbs, spices, and other flavor-enhancing techniques can add taste without excess sodium.

- **Avoiding High-Sodium Foods:** Limiting or avoiding high-sodium foods, such as processed meats, canned soups, and salty snacks, is essential for managing sodium intake.

- **Collaboration with Healthcare Providers:** Working with healthcare providers and registered dietitians ensures appropriate sodium intake based on individual health needs and kidney function.

By lowering sodium intake, individuals can support blood pressure control, preserve kidney function, and reduce the risk of cardiovascular and renal complications. Adopting a low-sodium dietary approach, along with other elements of a balanced diabetic renal diet, contributes to better diabetes and kidney management, leading to improved overall health and well-being.

2. Lowering Phosphorus

Lowering phosphorus intake is a crucial dietary strategy for individuals with kidney disease, as it helps support kidney function and prevent complications associated with elevated phosphorus levels.

- **Kidney Function Support:** The kidneys play a vital role in regulating phosphorus levels in the body. In kidney disease, the kidneys may struggle to remove excess phosphorus, leading to elevated levels (hyperphosphatemia). Reducing phosphorus intake eases the burden on the kidneys, slowing the progression of kidney damage.
- **Bone Health:** High phosphorus levels can lead to a mineral imbalance, causing the body to pull calcium from the bones. Over time, this can weaken bones and increase the risk of bone fractures. Lowering phosphorus intake helps maintain bone health.
- **Cardiovascular Health:** Elevated phosphorus levels are associated with an increased risk of cardiovascular complications, including heart

disease and calcification of blood vessels. Managing phosphorus intake supports overall cardiovascular well-being.

- **Reading Food Labels:** Monitoring phosphorus intake requires reading food labels to identify phosphorus-containing additives and preservatives. Choosing low-phosphorus alternatives is essential for individuals with kidney disease.
- **Limiting High-Phosphorus Foods:** Certain foods, including dairy products, nuts, seeds, and processed foods, are high in phosphorus. Lowering consumption of these foods helps control phosphorus levels.
- **Cooking and Meal Preparation:** Cooking techniques, such as leaching or soaking certain high-phosphorus foods, can reduce their phosphorus content. Careful meal preparation can help lower phosphorus intake.
- **Collaboration with Healthcare Providers:** Working with registered dietitians and healthcare providers ensures appropriate phosphorus intake based on individual kidney function and health needs.

By lowering phosphorus intake, individuals can support kidney health, maintain bone health, and reduce the risk of complications associated with kidney disease. Adopting a low-phosphorus dietary approach, combined with other elements of a balanced diabetic renal diet, contributes to effective diabetes and kidney management, promoting overall health and well-being.

3. Controlling Potassium

Controlling potassium intake is an essential dietary aspect for individuals with kidney disease, as it helps manage potassium levels in the body and prevents complications associated with hyperkalemia.

- **Kidney Function Support:** The kidneys play a critical role in regulating potassium levels in the body. In kidney disease, impaired kidney function can lead to high potassium levels (hyperkalemia). Controlling potassium intake eases the burden on the kidneys, supporting their function and reducing the risk of heart arrhythmias and other complications.
- **Cardiovascular Health:** High potassium levels can impact heart function, leading to irregular heartbeats and other cardiac issues. Managing potassium intake supports overall cardiovascular

health and reduces the risk of heart-related complications.

- **Reading Food Labels:** Monitoring potassium intake requires reading food labels to identify high-potassium foods. Choosing low-potassium alternatives is crucial for individuals with kidney disease.

- **Limiting High-Potassium Foods:** Certain foods, such as bananas, oranges, tomatoes, and potatoes, are high in potassium. Reducing consumption of these foods helps control potassium levels.

- **Cooking and Meal Preparation:** Cooking techniques, such as leaching or soaking certain high-potassium foods, can reduce their potassium content. Careful meal preparation can help lower potassium intake.

- **Medication Management:** Some medications, such as potassium-sparing diuretics, can increase potassium levels in the body. Managing medication intake in consultation with healthcare providers is essential for potassium control.

- **Collaboration with Healthcare Providers:** Working with registered dietitians and healthcare providers ensures appropriate potassium intake based on individual kidney function and health needs.

By controlling potassium intake, individuals can support kidney function, maintain cardiovascular health, and reduce the risk of complications associated with kidney disease. Adhering to a low-potassium dietary approach, combined with other elements of a balanced diabetic renal diet, contributes to effective diabetes and kidney management, promoting overall health and well-being.

4. Managing Carbohydrates

Managing carbohydrates is a fundamental aspect of diabetes management, as it directly impacts blood glucose levels. Individuals with diabetes must be mindful of their carbohydrate intake to achieve stable blood sugar levels and prevent complications.

- **Understanding Glycemic Index:** The glycemic index (GI) measures how quickly a carbohydrate-containing food raises blood glucose levels. Choosing low-GI foods, such as whole grains, legumes, and non-starchy vegetables, helps manage blood sugar by producing a gradual and steady rise.
- **Carbohydrate Counting:** Carbohydrate counting is a common method used by individuals with

diabetes to manage blood glucose levels. By tracking the total amount of carbohydrates consumed, individuals can adjust insulin doses or medication regimens accordingly.

- **Meal Planning:** Creating balanced and portion-controlled meals is essential for managing carbohydrates effectively. Distributing carbohydrates evenly throughout the day can help prevent blood sugar spikes.
- **Monitoring Blood Glucose:** Regularly monitoring blood glucose levels provides valuable insights into how different foods and meals affect blood sugar. This information helps individuals make informed decisions about their dietary choices.
- **Collaborating with Healthcare Providers:** Working with healthcare providers and registered dietitians is essential for personalized guidance on managing carbohydrates based on individual health needs and diabetes control goals.

By effectively managing carbohydrates, individuals with diabetes can achieve better blood glucose control, reduce the risk of complications, and improve overall well-being. A balanced approach to carbohydrate intake, combined with other elements of a well-rounded diabetic renal diet, contributes to successful diabetes management and enhanced quality of life.

E. Essential Nutrients for Diabetes and Kidney Health

1. Fiber

Fiber is a vital component of a well-balanced diabetic renal diet that supports both diabetes management and kidney health. Found in plant-based foods, fiber offers numerous health benefits and plays a significant role in overall well-being.

- **Blood Glucose Control:** Dietary fiber slows the absorption of glucose, leading to more gradual rises in blood sugar levels after meals. This helps individuals with diabetes maintain stable blood glucose levels, reducing the risk of spikes and hypoglycemia.
- **Digestive Health:** Fiber promotes healthy digestion by adding bulk to stool, preventing constipation, and supporting regular bowel movements. Adequate fiber intake can help prevent gastrointestinal issues and promote gut health.
- **Weight Management:** High-fiber foods are often low in calories and contribute to a feeling of

fullness. Including fiber-rich foods in the diet helps with weight management and portion control, reducing the risk of obesity-related complications in individuals with diabetes.

• **Heart Health:** Fiber has heart-protective properties, as it helps lower cholesterol levels and reduce the risk of cardiovascular disease, a common concern for individuals with diabetes.

• **Collaborating with Healthcare Providers:** Registered dietitians and healthcare providers can offer personalised recommendations on fiber intake based on individual health needs and diabetes management goals.

Incorporating fiber-rich foods, such as fruits, vegetables, whole grains, and legumes, into the diet supports blood glucose management, digestive health, weight control, and overall well-being. A well-balanced diabetic renal diet that includes adequate fiber contributes to effective diabetes and kidney management, leading to improved health outcomes and a higher quality of life.

2. Omega-3 Fatty Acids

Omega-3 fatty acids are essential nutrients with numerous health benefits, making them a valuable component of a diabetic renal diet that supports diabetes management and kidney health.

• **Heart Health:** Omega-3 fatty acids' potential to protect the heart has been well investigated. They help reduce triglyceride levels, lower blood pressure, and decrease the risk of cardiovascular disease, which is a common concern for individuals with diabetes.

• **Anti-Inflammatory Effects:** Omega-3 fatty acids exhibit anti-inflammatory properties, which can be beneficial for individuals with diabetes and kidney disease. Reducing inflammation may help alleviate symptoms and slow the progression of kidney damage.

• **Brain Health:** Omega-3 fatty acids are crucial for brain function and cognitive health. They play a role in maintaining brain cell membranes and supporting neurological well-being.

• **Immune System Support:** Omega-3 fatty acids contribute to a healthy immune system, enhancing the body's ability to fight off infections and illnesses.

• **Food Sources:** Omega-3 fatty acids can be found in fatty fish (e.g., flaxseeds, chia seeds, and walnuts), as well as sardines, mackerel, and salmon.

Incorporating these foods into the diet provides a natural source of these beneficial nutrients.

• **Collaboration with Healthcare Providers:** Working with registered dietitians and healthcare providers ensures appropriate omega-3 fatty acid intake based on individual health needs and kidney function.

By including omega-3 fatty acids in the diet, individuals can support heart health, reduce inflammation, and promote overall well-being. A balanced diabetic renal diet that incorporates these essential nutrients contributes to effective diabetes and kidney management, leading to improved health outcomes and a better quality of life.

3. Antioxidants

Antioxidants are essential compounds that play a crucial role in a well-rounded diabetic renal diet, supporting both diabetes management and kidney health. These powerful substances protect the body from oxidative stress, which can lead to cell damage and contribute to various health issues.

• **Cell Protection:** Antioxidants neutralise harmful molecules called free radicals, which are produced during normal metabolic processes and exposure to environmental factors. By neutralising free radicals, antioxidants safeguard cells from damage and help maintain their integrity.

• **Heart Health:** Antioxidants have been associated with improved heart health. They help reduce oxidative stress on blood vessels and prevent inflammation, which supports overall cardiovascular well-being.

• **Immune System Support:** Antioxidants boost the immune system by defending the body against infections and enhancing its ability to fight off illnesses.

• **Diabetic Complications:** For individuals with diabetes, antioxidants may help reduce the risk of diabetes-related complications, such as nerve damage and eye problems, by protecting cells from damage caused by elevated blood glucose levels.

• **Food Sources:** Antioxidants are found in a variety of fruits, vegetables, nuts, and seeds. Brightly coloured fruits and vegetables, such as berries, citrus fruits, and leafy greens, are particularly rich in these beneficial compounds.

• **Collaboration with Healthcare Providers:** Working with registered dietitians and healthcare providers ensures adequate antioxidant intake based on individual health needs and kidney function.

By incorporating antioxidant-rich foods into the diet, individuals can protect their cells, support heart health, and promote overall well-being. A balanced diabetic renal diet that includes a variety of antioxidant-rich foods contributes to effective diabetes and kidney management, leading to improved health outcomes and a higher quality of life.

4. Vitamin D

Vitamin D is a crucial fat-soluble vitamin that plays a significant role in a well-balanced diabetic renal diet, supporting both diabetes management and kidney health. It is essential for various bodily functions and overall well-being.

- **Bone Health:** Vitamin D is vital for calcium absorption and bone health. Adequate levels of vitamin D help maintain strong bones and reduce the risk of fractures and osteoporosis, especially important for individuals with kidney disease who may have impaired bone health.

• **Immune System Support:** Vitamin D plays a role in supporting the immune system, enhancing the body's ability to fight off infections and diseases.

• **Blood Glucose Control:** Emerging research suggests that vitamin D may play a role in improving insulin sensitivity and blood glucose control, potentially benefiting individuals with diabetes.

• **Cardiovascular Health:** Vitamin D is associated with cardiovascular health, as it helps reduce inflammation and support overall heart function.

• **Sunlight and Food Sources:** The body can produce vitamin D through exposure to sunlight. Additionally, it can be obtained from dietary sources such as fatty fish, fortified dairy products, and egg yolks.

• **Collaboration with Healthcare Providers:** Working with registered dietitians and healthcare providers ensures appropriate vitamin D intake based on individual health needs and kidney function.

By incorporating vitamin D-rich foods and ensuring adequate sunlight exposure, individuals can support bone health, immune function, and overall well-being. A balanced diabetic renal diet that includes sufficient vitamin D contributes to effective diabetes and kidney management, leading to improved health outcomes and a better quality of life.

F. Snacking and Beverages in the Diabetic Renal Diet

1. Nutrient-Dense Snacks

Nutrient-dense snacks are an essential part of a well-rounded diabetic renal diet, providing valuable nutrients without excess calories or harmful additives. These snacks offer a convenient and delicious way to support diabetes management and kidney health between meals.

• **Balanced Nutrition:** Nutrient-dense snacks provide a balanced combination of essential nutrients, such as vitamins, minerals, fiber, and healthy fats. They help maintain stable blood glucose levels and promote overall well-being.

• **Sustained Energy:** Snacking on nutrient-dense options can provide a steady source of energy throughout the day. This helps prevent energy dips and supports physical activity levels.

• **Portion Control:** Opting for nutrient-dense snacks encourages portion control, preventing overeating and aiding weight management, which is crucial for individuals with diabetes and kidney health concerns.

• **Blood Glucose Management:** Snacks with a low glycemic index, such as raw vegetables with hummus, nuts, or Greek yoghourt, can help manage blood glucose levels effectively and prevent blood sugar spikes.

• **Collaboration with Healthcare Providers:** Working with registered dietitians and healthcare providers ensures appropriate snack choices based on individual health needs and kidney function.

By incorporating nutrient-dense snacks into the diet, individuals can support blood glucose management, promote overall health, and enhance diabetes and kidney management. Smart snack choices, combined with other elements of a balanced diabetic renal diet, contribute to improved health outcomes and a better quality of life.

2. Hydration

Hydration is a fundamental aspect of a well-rounded diabetic renal diet that supports both diabetes management and kidney health. Staying adequately hydrated is crucial for maintaining overall well-being and supporting proper kidney function.

- **Kidney Health:** Adequate hydration is essential for the kidneys to effectively filter waste and toxins from the blood, producing urine to eliminate these substances from the body. Staying hydrated helps maintain kidney function, reducing the risk of kidney damage and kidney stones.

- **Blood Glucose Control:** Proper hydration supports stable blood glucose levels. Dehydration can lead to elevated blood sugar levels, as the kidneys may conserve fluid, resulting in higher glucose concentrations in the blood. Maintaining adequate fluid intake helps manage blood glucose and supports diabetes management.

- **Fluid Balance:** Proper hydration helps maintain a balanced fluid level in the body, preventing dehydration and overhydration. Maintaining a proper fluid balance is crucial for overall health and prevents potential complications associated with fluid imbalances.

- **Energy Levels:** Staying hydrated helps maintain energy levels, supporting physical activity and mental alertness.

- **Collaboration with Healthcare Providers:** Working with registered dietitians and healthcare providers ensures appropriate fluid intake based on individual health needs and kidney function.

By prioritising hydration, individuals can support kidney health, manage blood glucose levels, and promote overall well-being. Drinking enough fluids, especially water, is a simple yet powerful aspect of a well-balanced diabetic renal diet, contributing to effective diabetes and kidney management and leading to improved health outcomes and quality of life.

G. Meal Planning for Special Dietary Needs

1. Vegetarian and Vegan Diets

Vegetarian and vegan diets are dietary choices that exclude or minimise the consumption of animal products, respectively. These diets have gained popularity due to their potential health benefits and ethical or environmental considerations.

- **Health Benefits:** Well-planned vegetarian and vegan diets can be nutritionally rich, providing ample vitamins, minerals, and fiber. These diets are often associated with lower risks of heart disease, hypertension, and certain cancers, and they may support diabetes management and kidney health.
- **Weight Management:** Plant-based diets are generally lower in saturated fats and calories, making them helpful for weight management, which is particularly important for individuals with diabetes and kidney concerns.
- **Ethical and Environmental Impact:** Many people adopt vegetarian or vegan diets to align with their ethical beliefs, as these diets involve fewer animal products and may lead to reduced environmental impact.
- **Nutritional Considerations:** While vegetarian and vegan diets offer health benefits, individuals need to pay attention to certain nutrients, such as protein, vitamin B12, iron, and omega-3 fatty acids. Proper planning and supplementation, if necessary, are essential to meet nutritional needs.

- **Collaboration with Healthcare Providers:** Working with registered dietitians and healthcare providers ensures that vegetarian or vegan diets are tailored to individual health needs and support diabetes and kidney management.

By adopting well-balanced vegetarian or vegan diets, individuals can enjoy a diverse range of nutrient-rich plant-based foods, experience potential health benefits, and promote ethical and sustainable food choices. Proper planning and collaboration with healthcare providers contribute to successful diabetes and kidney management, leading to improved overall well-being and quality of life.

2. Gluten-Free Diet

A gluten-free diet is a dietary approach that eliminates gluten, a protein found in wheat, barley, rye, and their derivatives. This diet is essential for individuals with celiac disease or gluten sensitivity, as gluten consumption triggers an immune response, damaging the small intestine lining and leading to various health issues.

- **Celiac Disease Management:** A gluten-free diet is the only treatment for celiac disease. By avoiding gluten-containing foods, individuals with celiac disease can prevent intestinal damage and improve nutrient absorption.

- **Gluten Sensitivity:** Some individuals may experience gluten sensitivity, a condition where gluten consumption causes digestive discomfort and other symptoms. Adopting a gluten-free diet can relieve these signs and symptoms and enhance general health.

- **Diabetes and Gluten-Free Diet:** Some individuals with diabetes choose a gluten-free diet due to personal preferences or potential health benefits. However, it is essential to carefully monitor carbohydrate intake and food choices to maintain stable blood glucose levels.

- **Gluten-Free Substitutes:** A variety of gluten-free grains and flours, such as rice, corn, quinoa, and almond flour, are available as substitutes for traditional gluten-containing products.

- **Nutritional Considerations:** A well-planned gluten-free diet can be nutritionally adequate. However, individuals must ensure sufficient intake of nutrients like fiber, iron, calcium, and B vitamins by including gluten-free whole grains, fruits, vegetables, and fortified products.

- **Collaboration with Healthcare Providers:** Working with registered dietitians and healthcare providers ensures that a gluten-free diet meets individual health needs and supports diabetes and kidney management.

For individuals with celiac disease or gluten sensitivity, a well-managed gluten-free diet is crucial for preventing complications and promoting overall health. By selecting gluten-free options mindfully and collaborating with healthcare providers, individuals can successfully navigate a gluten-free diet while maintaining effective diabetes and kidney management.

3. Food Allergies and Intolerances

Food allergies and intolerances are conditions that involve adverse reactions to certain foods. Understanding and managing these conditions is vital for individuals with diabetes and kidney health concerns.

- **Food Allergies:** Food allergies trigger an immune response, leading to symptoms like hives, swelling, difficulty breathing, and in severe cases, anaphylaxis. The most typical allergies include dairy, eggs, nuts, and shellfish. Managing food allergies involves strict avoidance of the allergen and carrying emergency medication, like an epinephrine auto-injector, in case of accidental exposure.

- **Food Intolerances:** Food intolerances result from the body's inability to properly digest certain foods or components, leading to gastrointestinal symptoms like bloating, gas, and diarrhoea. Lactose intolerance is a common example. Managing food intolerances requires limiting or avoiding problematic foods and finding suitable alternatives.

- **Gluten Sensitivity:** Gluten sensitivity, different from celiac disease, may cause digestive discomfort and other symptoms when consuming gluten. A gluten-free diet is necessary for individuals with this sensitivity.

- **Cross-Contamination:** Individuals with food allergies must be vigilant about cross-contamination, which occurs when allergens come into contact with other foods during preparation or cooking. Proper food handling and communication with food service providers are essential.

- **Collaboration with Healthcare Providers:** Working with registered dietitians and healthcare providers helps identify food allergies and intolerances, and develop personalised meal plans that support diabetes and kidney management.

By identifying and managing food allergies and intolerances, individuals can prevent adverse reactions, promote better digestion, and support diabetes and kidney health. Collaborating with healthcare providers ensures safe and appropriate dietary choices, contributing to improved overall well-being and a higher quality of life.

H. Lifestyle Considerations and Diabetes Management

1. Physical Activity

Physical activity is a key component of a healthy lifestyle for individuals with diabetes and kidney health concerns. Regular exercise offers numerous benefits that support diabetes management, cardiovascular health, and overall well-being.

- **Weight Management:** Physical activity contributes to weight loss or maintenance, which is essential for individuals with diabetes and kidney concerns. Maintaining a healthy weight supports better blood glucose control and reduces the risk of diabetes-related complications.

- **Cardiovascular Health:** Regular exercise improves heart health by reducing blood pressure, cholesterol levels, and the risk of cardiovascular diseases. This is especially important for individuals with diabetes, who have a higher risk of heart-related issues.
- **Kidney Function:** Physical activity supports kidney health by promoting blood flow to the kidneys and reducing the risk of kidney damage.
- **Collaboration with Healthcare Providers:** Individuals with diabetes and kidney concerns should work with healthcare providers to develop safe and appropriate exercise plans that align with their health needs and goals.

By incorporating regular physical activity into their daily routines, individuals with diabetes and kidney health concerns can enjoy numerous health benefits, including improved blood glucose control, cardiovascular health, and overall well-being. Engaging in appropriate exercises, based on individual health needs, supports effective diabetes and kidney management, leading to improved health outcomes and a higher quality of life.

2. Blood Glucose Monitoring

Blood glucose monitoring is a critical practice for individuals with diabetes to manage their condition effectively. Regularly checking blood glucose levels provides valuable insights into how food, physical activity, and medication impact blood sugar levels.

- **Diabetes Management:** Blood glucose monitoring allows individuals to make informed decisions about their diabetes management. It helps track how well dietary choices, physical activity, and medications are controlling blood sugar levels.
- **Hypoglycemia and Hyperglycemia Detection:** Monitoring blood glucose levels helps identify and address episodes of low blood sugar (hypoglycemia) and high blood sugar (hyperglycemia) promptly. Prompt intervention can prevent serious complications.
- **Individualised Treatment:** Blood glucose data helps healthcare providers tailor individualised treatment plans, including medication adjustments and dietary recommendations.
- **Improved Diabetes Control:** Regular blood glucose monitoring is associated with improved

diabetes control and reduced risk of long-term complications.

• **Lifestyle Impact:** Blood glucose data reveals how lifestyle choices affect blood sugar levels, motivating individuals to make healthier choices and maintain a balanced diabetic renal diet.

• **Collaboration with Healthcare Providers:** Working with healthcare providers and diabetes educators ensures appropriate blood glucose monitoring practices and empowers individuals to manage their condition effectively.

By monitoring blood glucose levels regularly, individuals with diabetes can make informed decisions about their daily activities and treatments, leading to better blood sugar control and overall diabetes management. It is an essential tool in supporting a well-balanced diabetic renal diet and contributes to improved health outcomes and a higher quality of life.

3. Medication Adherence

Adhering to prescribed medications, including medications for diabetes and blood pressure management, is essential for overall health and disease management.

- **Cardiovascular Health:** Proper medication adherence can support heart health by managing blood pressure, cholesterol levels, and reducing the risk of cardiovascular complications.
- **Preventing Complications:** Following medication regimens helps prevent or delay diabetes-related complications, such as nerve damage, eye problems, and cardiovascular diseases.
- **Collaboration with Healthcare Providers:** Engaging with healthcare providers and discussing any challenges related to medication adherence helps develop strategies to improve compliance and address any concerns.
- **Lifestyle Impact:** Medication adherence complements other aspects of diabetes and kidney management, such as diet, exercise, and regular check-ups.

By adhering to prescribed medications, individuals can effectively manage diabetes and kidney health, leading to improved overall well-being and a higher quality of life. Consistent medication use, in conjunction with other aspects of diabetes and kidney management, contributes to better health outcomes and empowers individuals to take an active role in their health journey.

4. Blood Pressure Control

Blood pressure control is a vital aspect of managing both diabetes and kidney health. High blood pressure, also known as hypertension, is a common complication of diabetes and can worsen kidney damage over time. Proper blood pressure management offers several benefits:

- **Kidney Health:** High blood pressure can damage blood vessels in the kidneys, leading to reduced kidney function. Controlling blood pressure helps preserve kidney health and slows the progression of kidney disease.
- **Cardiovascular Health:** Hypertension is a significant risk factor for heart disease, stroke, and other cardiovascular complications. Blood pressure control reduces the risk of these serious conditions.
- **Diabetes Management:** Maintaining normal blood pressure levels complements diabetes management, as it lowers the risk of diabetes-related complications and contributes to stable blood glucose control.

- **Lifestyle Modifications:** Lifestyle changes, including adopting a balanced diabetic renal diet, regular physical activity, and stress reduction, play a vital role in blood pressure control.
- **Medication Management:** For some individuals, medications may be necessary to achieve optimal blood pressure levels. Adhering to prescribed medications, as directed by healthcare providers, is crucial for successful blood pressure control.
- **Collaboration with Healthcare Providers:** Regular blood pressure monitoring and working closely with healthcare providers help identify the most appropriate treatment plan for each individual's needs.

By actively managing blood pressure, individuals can reduce the risk of kidney and cardiovascular complications associated with diabetes. A comprehensive approach that includes lifestyle modifications and medication adherence, in consultation with healthcare providers, contributes to effective blood pressure control and improved overall health and well-being.

5. Smoking Cessation

Smoking cessation is a critical step in managing both diabetes and kidney health. Smoking is a major risk factor for various health issues, and quitting offers significant benefits for individuals with these conditions.

• **Cardiovascular Health:** Smoking damages blood vessels, leading to an increased risk of heart disease and stroke. Quitting smoking improves cardiovascular health and reduces the risk of related complications, which is especially important for individuals with diabetes.

• **Kidney Health:** Smoking harms blood vessels in the kidneys, exacerbating kidney damage and worsening kidney function. Quitting smoking can slow the progression of kidney disease and protect kidney health.

• **Blood Glucose Control:** Smoking affects insulin sensitivity and glucose metabolism, making blood glucose control more challenging for individuals with diabetes. Smoking cessation can contribute to better blood glucose management.

• **Respiratory Health:** Smoking damages the lungs and worsens respiratory conditions, increasing the risk of infections and complications. Quitting smoking supports respiratory health and reduces the risk of respiratory issues.

• **Collaborating with Healthcare Providers:** Working with healthcare providers and smoking cessation programs provides valuable support and resources to quit smoking successfully.

• **Quality of Life:** Smoking cessation improves overall well-being, energy levels, and lung function, leading to a better quality of life for individuals with diabetes and kidney health concerns.

By quitting smoking, individuals can significantly improve their health outcomes, reduce the risk of complications, and enhance their overall well-being. It is a vital step in managing diabetes and kidney health effectively, leading to improved health outcomes and a higher quality of life.

6. Stress Management

Stress management is an essential aspect of diabetes and kidney health management, as chronic stress can negatively impact blood glucose levels and overall well-being. Adopting effective stress management techniques offers several benefits:

- **Blood Glucose Control:** High levels of stress can lead to hormonal imbalances and increase blood glucose levels. Managing stress helps stabilise blood sugar levels and supports diabetes management.

- **Cardiovascular Health:** Chronic stress can raise blood pressure and contribute to heart disease, a common concern for individuals with diabetes. Stress management promotes better cardiovascular health and reduces the risk of related complications.

Immune Function: Prolonged stress impairs immunity, leaving people more prone to illnesses. Stress management supports immune function and overall health.

- **Coping Skills:** Learning healthy coping strategies helps individuals navigate life's challenges without resorting to unhealthy habits, such as emotional eating or smoking.

- **Sleep Quality:** Stress can disrupt sleep patterns, impacting overall health and exacerbating diabetes management. Managing stress improves sleep quality, leading to better overall well-being.

- **Collaboration with Healthcare Providers:** Working with healthcare providers and counsellors provides personalised guidance and support in adopting stress management techniques.

By incorporating stress management practices, such as exercise, mindfulness, deep breathing, and relaxation techniques, individuals can improve their diabetes and kidney health management. Reducing stress levels contributes to better blood glucose control, cardiovascular health, and overall well-being, leading to improved health outcomes and a higher quality of life.

I. Meal Planning and Eating Out

1. Meal Prepping

Meal prepping is a practical and beneficial approach to managing both diabetes and kidney health. It involves planning and preparing meals in advance, ensuring healthier food choices, portion control, and consistent adherence to a balanced diabetic renal diet.

- **Time Efficiency:** Meal prepping saves time during busy days, as meals are already prepared and can be easily reheated or assembled. This reduces the temptation to opt for less healthy fast food choices.
- **Portion Control:** Preparing meals in advance allows for portion control, which is crucial for

individuals with diabetes to manage blood glucose levels and support weight management.

● **Nutrient-Rich Choices:** Meal prepping facilitates the inclusion of nutrient-rich ingredients, such as fruits, vegetables, lean proteins, and whole grains, supporting diabetes and kidney health.

● **Budget-Friendly:** By planning meals in advance and buying ingredients in bulk, meal prepping can be cost-effective, reducing food waste and unnecessary spending.

● **Consistency:** Regularly prepping meals encourages a consistent eating pattern, promoting better blood glucose control and overall health.

● **Collaboration with Healthcare Providers:** Working with registered dietitians and healthcare providers ensures meal plans align with individual health needs and diabetes and kidney management goals.

By adopting meal prepping, individuals can make healthier food choices, manage portion sizes, and maintain consistent eating habits, leading to improved blood glucose control, kidney health, and overall well-being. It is a valuable tool in supporting effective diabetes and kidney management and contributes to better health outcomes and a higher quality of life.

2. Eating Out

Eating out can be enjoyable and manageable for individuals with diabetes and kidney health concerns, with some thoughtful planning and smart choices.

- **Menu Selection:** Look for restaurants with diverse menu options, including salads, grilled proteins, and vegetable-based dishes. Avoid high-sodium and high-sugar items.
- **Portion Control:** Be mindful of portion sizes, as restaurants often serve larger servings. Take into account splitting the meal or taking half home for later.
- **Customization:** Don't hesitate to ask for modifications, such as opting for whole-grain bread or requesting sauce on the side to control sodium intake.
- **Beverage Choices:** Opt for water, unsweetened tea, or low-calorie options to avoid excessive sugar and calorie intake.
- **Pre-planning:** Check online menus before going out to make informed choices, and consider eating a

small, balanced snack beforehand to avoid overeating.

• **Dietary Restrictions:** Inform the server about any dietary restrictions or food allergies to ensure a safe and enjoyable dining experience.

• **Collaboration with Healthcare Providers:** Discuss eating out strategies with healthcare providers or dietitians to receive personalised advice and support.

With mindful choices and pre-planning, eating out can be a delicious and health-conscious experience. Smart decisions and collaboration with healthcare providers contribute to effective diabetes and kidney management, leading to improved health outcomes and a higher quality of life.

J. The Role of Support and Education

1. Diabetes Education Programs

Diabetes education programs are invaluable resources for individuals with diabetes and kidney health concerns. These programs offer comprehensive and evidence-based information, empowering individuals to manage their condition effectively and improve their overall well-being.

- **Knowledge and Skills:** Diabetes education programs provide essential knowledge about diabetes management, blood glucose monitoring, healthy eating, physical activity, and medication adherence. They equip individuals with the skills needed to make informed decisions about their health.

- **Personalised Guidance:** These programs offer personalised guidance, taking into account individual health needs, lifestyle, and preferences. Healthcare professionals work closely with participants to develop tailored diabetes management plans.

 Support and Motivation: Diabetes education programs create a supportive environment where individuals can share experiences, seek guidance, and receive encouragement. This support fosters motivation to adopt healthier habits and overcome challenges.

- **Preventing Complications:** Education programs emphasise the importance of regular check-ups, blood glucose control, and lifestyle modifications to prevent or delay diabetes-related complications.

- **Collaboration with Healthcare Providers:** These programs involve collaboration with healthcare providers, dietitians, diabetes educators, and other experts to provide well-rounded support and guidance.

• **Long-Term Success:** Diabetes education programs focus on empowering individuals to manage their condition independently, promoting long-term success in diabetes and kidney health management.

By participating in diabetes education programs, individuals gain valuable tools, support, and knowledge to effectively manage their condition. These programs contribute to improved blood glucose control, better kidney health, and enhanced overall well-being, leading to better health outcomes and a higher quality of life.

2. Support Groups

Support groups play a crucial role in helping individuals with diabetes and kidney health concerns cope with their condition, providing emotional support, valuable information, and a sense of community.

• **Emotional Support:** Support groups offer a safe space for individuals to share their experiences, challenges, and emotions related to living with diabetes and kidney health concerns. This emotional support can alleviate feelings of isolation and anxiety.

- **Shared Knowledge:** Participants in support groups can exchange information and insights about managing diabetes and kidney health effectively. Learning from others' experiences can be valuable in making informed decisions about one's own health.

- **Coping Strategies:** Support groups provide opportunities to learn coping strategies for handling stress, managing blood glucose levels, and overcoming barriers to a healthy lifestyle.

- **Empowerment:** By participating in support groups, individuals feel empowered to take an active role in managing their health and making positive changes.

- **Motivation:** Seeing others overcome challenges and achieve health goals can be motivating and inspiring, encouraging individuals to stay committed to their diabetes and kidney health management.

- **Sense of Community:** Support groups create a sense of belonging and understanding, fostering connections with others who share similar experiences.

By joining support groups, individuals with diabetes and kidney health concerns can find understanding, encouragement, and practical advice. This sense of community and support contributes to better diabetes and kidney management, improved mental well-being, and an enhanced quality of life.

In Summary

Navigating a diabetic renal diet is a complex yet crucial undertaking for individuals managing both diabetes and kidney health. Understanding the principles of the diet, creating personalised meal plans, adapting recipes, and addressing individual dietary needs are essential components of a successful diabetic renal diet. By adhering to the key principles and collaborating with healthcare providers, individuals can effectively manage blood glucose levels, support kidney health, and reduce the risk of diabetes-related complications. A well-balanced and nutrient-rich diabetic renal diet, combined with regular physical activity and adherence to prescribed medications, contributes to overall well-being and enhanced quality of life for individuals navigating the challenges of diabetes and kidney health. Proactive education, support, and lifestyle modifications play a pivotal role in optimising outcomes and empowering individuals to take control of their health journey.

Chapter Three

The Power of Nutrient-Rich Ingredients: Enhancing Diabetes and Kidney Health

The role of nutrition in managing diabetes and kidney health cannot be overstated. Consuming nutrient-rich ingredients is key to supporting blood glucose control, kidney function, and overall well-being for individuals with these health concerns.

In this comprehensive guide, we will explore the power of nutrient-rich ingredients and their impact on diabetes and kidney health.

A. Understanding Nutrient-Rich Ingredients

Nutrient-rich ingredients refer to foods that are packed with essential vitamins, minerals, fiber, and other beneficial compounds while being relatively low in calories and harmful additives. These ingredients provide the necessary nutrients for optimal body function and play a significant role in supporting diabetes and kidney health.

Benefits of Nutrient-Rich Ingredients

The benefits of incorporating nutrient-rich ingredients into the diet are numerous and far-reaching. They include:
- Supporting blood glucose control and diabetes management
- Promoting kidney health and preventing kidney damage
- Enhancing cardiovascular health and reducing the risk of heart-related complications
- Providing essential nutrients for overall well-being and maintaining a healthy weight

Types of Nutrient-Rich Ingredients

Various types of nutrient-rich ingredients are essential for diabetes and kidney health management. These include:
- **Fruits and vegetables:** Rich in vitamins, minerals, antioxidants, and fiber.
- **Whole grains:** Providing complex carbohydrates, fiber, and essential nutrients.

- **Lean proteins:** Supporting muscle health and providing amino acids for bodily functions.
- **Healthy fats:** Beneficial for heart health and the absorption of fat-soluble vitamins.

B. Nutrient-Rich Ingredients and Diabetes Management

Effective diabetes management revolves around controlling blood glucose levels and making healthier food choices. Nutrient-rich ingredients play a vital role in achieving these goals and offer unique benefits for individuals with diabetes.

1. Impact on Blood Glucose Control

Nutrient-rich ingredients, particularly those with a low glycemic index, help stabilise blood glucose levels and prevent spikes. These ingredients include:
- **Non-starchy vegetables:** Leafy greens, broccoli, cauliflower, and bell peppers.
- **Berries:** Blueberries, strawberries, raspberries, and blackberries.
- **Legumes:** Lentils, chickpeas, and kidney beans.

2. Supporting Weight Management

Supporting weight management is a critical aspect of diabetes and kidney health management. For individuals with diabetes, maintaining a healthy weight is essential for stable blood glucose control and reducing the risk of complications. For those with kidney health concerns, weight management is crucial to ease the burden on the kidneys and improve overall health.

Incorporating nutrient-rich ingredients into the diet plays a key role in supporting weight management. These ingredients are typically low in calories but high in essential nutrients and fiber, promoting satiety and reducing the risk of overeating. Including a variety of fruits, vegetables, whole grains, and lean proteins in meals helps individuals feel fuller for longer and control their caloric intake.

In addition to nutrient-rich ingredients, portion control and mindful eating practices are essential. Being aware of portion sizes and eating slowly to savor each bite can prevent overeating and support weight management goals.

Regular physical activity also plays a significant role in weight management. Engaging in regular exercise helps burn calories, maintain muscle mass, and improve overall fitness, contributing to a healthy weight.

By adopting a balanced diet rich in nutrient-dense ingredients, practising portion control, and incorporating physical activity into daily routines, individuals can effectively support weight management and positively impact diabetes and kidney health.

3. Glycemic Load and Carbohydrate Management

Glycemic load and carbohydrate management are crucial aspects of diabetes and kidney health management. Monitoring the glycemic load of foods and managing carbohydrate intake helps individuals maintain stable blood glucose levels and supports overall health.

Glycemic load refers to the amount of carbohydrates in a serving of food and its impact on blood glucose levels. Foods with a low glycemic load cause slower and more gradual increases in blood glucose levels, while those with a high glycemic load cause rapid spikes.

Managing carbohydrate intake is vital for individuals with diabetes because carbohydrates have the most significant impact on blood glucose levels. Glucose is created from carbohydrates and delivered into the bloodstream. By controlling carbohydrate consumption, individuals can better manage their blood glucose levels and reduce the risk of hyperglycemia.

Balancing carbohydrate intake with other macronutrients, such as protein and healthy fats, is essential for optimal blood glucose control and overall nutrition. Including nutrient-rich carbohydrates, such as whole grains, legumes, and non-starchy vegetables, in the diet can provide essential nutrients, fiber, and sustained energy without causing rapid spikes in blood glucose levels. By understanding glycemic load and managing carbohydrate intake, individuals can take proactive steps in diabetes and kidney health management. Making informed food choices, practising portion control, and collaborating with healthcare providers and dietitians contribute to effective carbohydrate management and support overall well-being.

C. Nutrient-Rich Ingredients and Kidney Health

For individuals with kidney health concerns, consuming nutrient-rich ingredients helps protect kidney function, maintain fluid balance, and reduce the risk of kidney damage.

1. Reducing Sodium Intake

Reducing sodium intake is vital for individuals with diabetes and kidney health concerns. High sodium consumption can lead to fluid retention, elevated blood pressure, and worsen kidney function. By adopting a low-sodium diet, individuals can support their overall health and reduce the risk of complications.

Processed and packaged foods are often high in sodium, so opting for fresh, whole foods is essential. Incorporating nutrient-rich ingredients, such as fruits, vegetables, and lean proteins, can help lower sodium intake while providing essential nutrients.

Reading food labels is crucial to identify high-sodium products and make informed choices. Choosing low-sodium or sodium-free alternatives can significantly impact sodium intake.

Cooking at home allows individuals to control the amount of salt used in their meals. Using herbs, spices, and other flavorings can enhance the taste of dishes without relying on excessive salt.

Collaborating with healthcare providers and registered dietitians to develop a personalized low-sodium meal plan is highly beneficial. These professionals can provide guidance, monitor sodium intake, and ensure that the diet aligns with individual health needs and goals.

By reducing sodium intake through mindful food choices, cooking practices, and collaboration with healthcare providers, individuals can promote kidney health, manage blood pressure, and support overall well-being.

2. Potassium and Phosphorus Management

Potassium and phosphorus management are critical considerations for individuals with kidney health concerns. Both minerals play essential roles in the body, but individuals with kidney issues need to monitor their intake to prevent imbalances and maintain kidney function.

I. Potassium Management:

Potassium is essential for nerve function, muscle contractions, and maintaining heart health. However, for those with kidney problems, excess potassium can lead to hyperkalemia, a condition characterised by high levels of potassium in the blood.

To manage potassium intake, individuals should limit high-potassium foods like bananas, oranges, potatoes, and tomatoes. Instead, they can incorporate lower-potassium options such as apples, berries, cucumbers, and rice.

II. Phosphorus Management:

Phosphorus is vital for bone health and various cellular functions. However, elevated phosphorus levels, known as hyperphosphatemia, can occur in kidney disease, leading to bone and cardiovascular complications.

To manage phosphorus intake, individuals should reduce consumption of phosphorus-rich foods, including dairy products, nuts, and processed foods containing phosphate additives. Opting for phosphorus-free or low-phosphorus alternatives can help maintain phosphorus balance.

Working with healthcare providers and registered dietitians is essential for creating personalised meal plans that effectively manage potassium and phosphorus levels while supporting overall kidney health and well-being. By being mindful of potassium and phosphorus sources in the diet, individuals can promote optimal kidney function and reduce the risk of related complications.

3. Promoting Fluid Balance

Promoting fluid balance is crucial for individuals with diabetes and kidney health concerns. Proper fluid management helps maintain hydration, supports kidney function, and prevents complications such as fluid overload and dehydration.

I. Adequate Fluid Intake:
Staying hydrated is essential for overall health, including kidney function and blood glucose control. Individuals should aim to consume an adequate amount of fluids daily, primarily through water, to support fluid balance.

II. Monitoring Fluid Intake:
For individuals with kidney health concerns, monitoring fluid intake is crucial, especially if kidney function is compromised. Following healthcare providers' recommendations on fluid intake helps prevent fluid retention and supports proper kidney function.

III. Limiting Fluids with High Sodium Content:
Fluids with a high sodium content can lead to fluid retention and worsen blood pressure and kidney function. Reducing the intake of high-sodium

beverages like sodas, sports drinks, and certain fruit juices is essential for promoting fluid balance.

IV. Managing Fluids with Diuretic Effects:

Some fluids, such as caffeine-containing beverages and alcoholic drinks, act as diuretics, increasing urine output and potentially affecting fluid balance. Moderating the consumption of such fluids is advisable.

V. Collaboration with Healthcare Providers:

Working closely with healthcare providers and registered dietitians helps individuals develop personalised fluid management strategies that align with their specific health needs and goals.

By promoting fluid balance through adequate hydration, monitoring fluid intake, and making mindful choices about fluid sources, individuals can support their kidney health, manage blood glucose levels, and promote overall well-being. Proper fluid management is a key aspect of diabetes and kidney health management, contributing to improved health outcomes and a higher quality of life.

D. Incorporating Nutrient-Rich Ingredients into the Diet

Integrating nutrient-rich ingredients into the diet can be achieved through a balanced approach, focusing on meal planning, portion control, and creative recipes.

1. Meal Planning

Meal planning is a fundamental tool for individuals with diabetes and kidney health concerns. It involves proactively organising and preparing meals in advance, offering numerous benefits for effective management of these conditions.

I. Blood Glucose Control: Meal planning allows individuals to incorporate nutrient-rich ingredients with a low glycemic index, helping stabilise blood glucose levels and preventing spikes after meals.

II. Portion Control: Planning meals in advance helps with portion control, ensuring appropriate serving sizes that support weight management and prevent overeating.

III. Nutrient-Rich Choices: With meal planning, individuals can prioritise nutrient-rich ingredients such as fruits, vegetables, whole grains, and lean proteins, ensuring a well-balanced diet that supports overall health.

IV. Sodium and Phosphorus Management: Individuals with kidney health concerns can control sodium and phosphorus intake by selecting low-sodium and low-phosphorus ingredients, reducing the risk of complications.

V. Time Efficiency: Meal planning saves time during busy days, as meals are already prepared or can be quickly assembled, reducing the likelihood of opting for less healthy fast food choices.

VI. Collaboration with Healthcare Providers: Working with healthcare providers and registered dietitians ensures meal plans align with individual health needs, providing personalised guidance for effective diabetes and kidney health management.

By adopting meal planning practices, individuals can take charge of their health, support blood glucose control and kidney health, and improve overall well-being. It is a valuable strategy for successful diabetes and kidney management, leading to improved health outcomes and a higher quality of life.

2. Portion Control

Portion control is a fundamental aspect of diabetes and kidney health management. It involves being mindful of the amount of food consumed during meals and snacks to maintain a balanced diet and support overall well-being.

I. Blood Glucose Control: Proper portion control helps regulate carbohydrate intake, preventing significant spikes in blood glucose levels after meals and promoting stable blood sugar control.

II. Weight Management: Monitoring portion sizes aids in managing caloric intake, supporting weight management, and reducing the risk of obesity-related complications.

III. Sodium and Phosphorus Management: For individuals with kidney health concerns, portion control assists in limiting the intake of high-sodium and high-phosphorus foods, promoting kidney health and preventing complications.

IV. Nutrient Intake: By controlling portion sizes, individuals can ensure they receive adequate nutrients from a variety of food groups without overconsumption, supporting overall health.

V. Mindful Eating: Practising portion control encourages mindful eating, promoting awareness of hunger and fullness cues and reducing the risk of overeating.

VI. Collaboration with Healthcare Providers: Healthcare providers and registered dietitians can offer personalised guidance on appropriate portion sizes based on individual health needs and goals.

By implementing portion control strategies, individuals can make informed food choices, achieve better blood glucose control, and support kidney health. It is a simple yet powerful tool in diabetes and kidney health management, contributing to improved health outcomes and a higher quality of life.

3. Nutrient-Rich Recipes

Nutrient-rich recipes are essential for individuals with diabetes and kidney health concerns, as they offer delicious and healthful options that support overall well-being. These recipes are centred around incorporating nutrient-dense ingredients, providing essential vitamins, minerals, and other beneficial compounds without excessive calories or harmful additives.

I. Balanced Nutritional Profile: Nutrient-rich recipes prioritise a balance of macronutrients and essential nutrients, such as fiber, vitamins, and antioxidants. They promote stable blood glucose levels and support kidney function.

II. Whole Foods Focus: These recipes often feature whole, unprocessed foods like fruits, vegetables, whole grains, and lean proteins, providing the body with essential nutrients without unnecessary additives.

III. Flavorful and Satisfying: Nutrient-rich recipes emphasise bold flavours and creative combinations, making meals enjoyable and satisfying while supporting portion control and overall health.

IV. Variety and Adaptability: These recipes offer versatility, allowing individuals to adapt them to their dietary preferences and needs, making them suitable for different tastes and health concerns.

V. Collaboration with Healthcare Providers: Working with healthcare providers and dietitians can help individuals develop personalised nutrient-rich recipes that align with their specific health needs and goals.

By incorporating nutrient-rich recipes into their meal planning, individuals can make healthy and enjoyable food choices, effectively manage diabetes and kidney health, and promote overall well-being. Nutrient-rich recipes offer a practical and tasty approach to better health outcomes and a higher quality of life.

E. Collaboration with Healthcare Providers and Dietitians

Collaboration with healthcare providers and dietitians is a critical component of managing diabetes and kidney health effectively. These professionals offer specialised expertise and guidance, providing valuable support to individuals with these health concerns.

I. Personalised Care: Healthcare providers and dietitians create personalised treatment plans that consider each individual's unique health needs, lifestyle, and preferences, tailoring interventions for optimal outcomes.

II. Nutritional Guidance: Dietitians play a pivotal role in developing balanced meal plans, incorporating nutrient-rich ingredients, managing portion sizes, and ensuring adequate nutrient intake to support diabetes and kidney health.

III. Blood Glucose Monitoring: Healthcare providers monitor blood glucose levels and interpret results to assess treatment effectiveness, making necessary adjustments to medication or lifestyle modifications.

IV. Medication Management: Healthcare providers closely monitor medications for diabetes and kidney health, adjusting dosages and prescribing additional therapies as needed to ensure optimal health outcomes.

V. Lifestyle Modifications: Collaborating with healthcare providers helps individuals implement sustainable lifestyle changes, such as regular physical activity, stress management, and smoking cessation, which significantly impact diabetes and kidney health.

VI. Preventive Care: Regular check-ups with healthcare providers and dietitians facilitate early detection of potential complications, enabling proactive intervention to prevent further health issues.

By working closely with healthcare providers and dietitians, individuals can gain a deeper understanding of their conditions, receive personalised guidance, and access essential resources for diabetes and kidney health management. This collaboration empowers individuals to take an active role in their health, leading to improved health outcomes and an enhanced quality of life.

In Summary

The power of nutrient-rich ingredients in enhancing diabetes and kidney health cannot be overlooked. Incorporating fruits, vegetables, whole grains, lean proteins, and healthy fats into the diet offers a multitude of benefits, supporting blood glucose control, kidney function, and overall well-being. By understanding the impact of nutrient-rich ingredients on diabetes and kidney health and collaborating with healthcare providers, individuals can take proactive steps to manage their conditions effectively and improve their quality of life.

Chapter Four

Breakfast Delights for Blood Sugar Control: Nourishing and Delicious Choices for a Healthy Start

Breakfast is considered the most important meal of the day, especially for individuals with diabetes. A balanced breakfast that includes nutrient-rich ingredients and supports blood sugar control is essential for managing diabetes effectively. In this comprehensive guide, we will explore various breakfast delights that not only tantalise the taste buds but also promote stable blood glucose levels for a healthy start to the day.

1. Understanding Blood Sugar Control

Understanding blood sugar control is essential for individuals with diabetes. The quantity of sugar in the blood is referred to as blood sugar, sometimes known as blood glucose. For individuals with diabetes, the body struggles to regulate blood sugar levels effectively, leading to fluctuations that can be harmful.

Maintaining stable blood sugar levels is critical to prevent complications and promote overall health. High blood sugar, known as hyperglycemia, can damage blood vessels, nerves, and organs over time. On the other hand, low blood sugar, known as hypoglycemia, can lead to dizziness, weakness, and confusion.

Monitoring blood sugar levels regularly, following a balanced diet that includes nutrient-rich ingredients with a low glycemic index, staying physically active, and taking medications as prescribed are essential components of blood sugar control for individuals with diabetes. By understanding and managing blood sugar effectively, individuals can significantly improve their diabetes management and enhance their overall well-being.

2. The Role of Nutrient-Rich Ingredients

Nutrient-rich ingredients play a crucial role in promoting overall health and well-being. These ingredients are packed with essential vitamins, minerals, antioxidants, and other beneficial compounds while being relatively low in calories and harmful additives.

Here are some key aspects of their role:

I. Supporting Nutritional Needs: Nutrient-rich ingredients provide a wide array of essential nutrients necessary for optimal body function. They supply vitamins, such as vitamin C and vitamin A, minerals like potassium and magnesium, and other micronutrients that support various physiological processes.

II. Blood Sugar Control: For individuals with diabetes, nutrient-rich ingredients with a low glycemic index are particularly beneficial. These ingredients, such as non-starchy vegetables, whole grains, and certain fruits, help stabilise blood glucose levels and prevent sharp spikes after meals.

III. Promoting Heart Health: Many nutrient-rich ingredients, such as oily fish rich in omega-3 fatty acids and nuts containing healthy fats, support cardiovascular health by reducing inflammation and improving cholesterol levels.

IV. Supporting Immune Function: Nutrient-rich ingredients, especially those rich in vitamin C, vitamin D, and zinc, help strengthen the immune system, reducing the risk of infections and supporting overall immunity.

V. Enhancing Digestive Health: High-fiber nutrient-rich ingredients, like fruits, vegetables, and whole grains, promote healthy digestion, prevent constipation, and support gut health.

VI. Weight Management: Nutrient-rich ingredients contribute to satiety, helping individuals feel full and satisfied, which can aid in weight management and prevent overeating.

VII. Reducing the Risk of Chronic Diseases: A diet rich in nutrient-dense ingredients is associated with a reduced risk of chronic diseases, such as type 2 diabetes, hypertension, and certain cancers.

By incorporating nutrient-rich ingredients into daily meals, individuals can create a balanced and nourishing diet that supports overall health and contributes to the prevention and management of various health conditions. Prioritising nutrient-rich foods ensures that the body receives the essential nutrients it needs for optimal functioning and well-being.

3. Creating Balanced Breakfasts

Creating balanced breakfasts is essential for starting the day on a nourishing and energising note. A well-balanced breakfast includes a mix of macronutrients, namely carbohydrates, proteins, and healthy fats, along with nutrient-rich ingredients to support overall health.

Here are some key principles for crafting balanced breakfasts:

I. Carbohydrates for Energy: Incorporate complex carbohydrates like whole grains, oats, or whole wheat products to provide sustained energy throughout the morning.

II. Protein for Satiety: Include a source of lean protein such as eggs, Greek yoghourt, or nuts, which helps promote feelings of fullness and prevents overeating.

III. Healthy Fats for Nutrient Absorption: Add healthy fats from sources like avocados, nuts, or seeds, which aid in the absorption of fat-soluble vitamins and provide satiety.

IV. Nutrient-Rich Ingredients: Include fruits, vegetables, and other nutrient-dense foods that supply essential vitamins, minerals, and antioxidants.

V. Mindful Portion Control: Be mindful of portion sizes to prevent excessive caloric intake and maintain blood sugar levels.

VI. Low-Glycemic Choices: Opt for low-glycemic index foods like berries, apples, or whole grains, which help regulate blood glucose levels.

Examples of balanced breakfasts:
- Oatmeal topped with sliced bananas, almonds, and a dollop of Greek yoghourt.
- Whole grain toast with avocado, poached eggs, and a side of mixed berries.
- Smoothie made with spinach, berries, almond milk, chia seeds, and a scoop of protein powder.

By following these guidelines, individuals can create breakfasts that provide sustained energy, promote satiety, support blood sugar control, and deliver essential nutrients for a healthy start to the day. Customising breakfast choices based on individual preferences and dietary needs ensures a balanced and enjoyable morning meal.

1. Preparing Whole Grain Wonders: Delicious and Nutritious Breakfast Options

Whole grains are a powerhouse of nutrients, offering a variety of health benefits and supporting blood sugar control.

Here are some creative and nutritious ways to incorporate whole grains into your breakfast:

- Overnight Oats:

Combine 1/2 cup rolled oats, 1 cup almond milk, a dash of cinnamon, and a spoonful of chia seeds in a jar.

Mix well and refrigerate overnight.

In the morning, top with sliced bananas, a sprinkle of nuts, and a drizzle of honey for added sweetness.

- Quinoa Breakfast Bowl:

Cook 1/2 cup quinoa in water or milk according to package instructions.

Stir in a handful of mixed berries, chopped nuts, and a drizzle of pure maple syrup.

Serve warm for a hearty and protein-packed breakfast.

- Whole Grain Pancakes:
In a bowl, mix 1 cup whole wheat flour, 1 tablespoon baking powder, 1 tablespoon sugar (optional), and a pinch of salt.
Add 1 cup almond milk and 1 tablespoon melted butter or oil.
On a nonstick pan, cook spoonfuls of the batter until golden brown on both sides.
Serve with Greek yoghurt and fresh fruit on the side.

- Brown Rice Porridge:
Cook 1/2 cup brown rice in water until tender.
Stir in a splash of almond milk, a handful of dried fruits, and a sprinkle of cinnamon.
Simmer until the mixture thickens, then serve warm with a handful of nuts on top.

- Whole Grain Breakfast Burrito:
Fill a whole-grain tortilla with scrambled eggs, sautéed vegetables, and black beans.
Add a sprinkle of shredded cheese and a dollop of avocado for a satisfying and protein-rich breakfast.

- Whole Grain Muffins:

Bake a batch of whole grain muffins with your choice of ingredients, such as blueberries, apples, or nuts.

Enjoy these portable breakfast treats with a side of fresh fruit.

- Whole Grain Cereal Bowl:

Choose a whole-grain cereal that is low in added sugars and high in fiber.

Mix it with your favorite milk or yogurt and add sliced bananas, strawberries, or a handful of raisins for extra flavor.

These whole grain wonders are not only delicious but also provide essential nutrients, fiber, and sustained energy to start your day right.

Experiment with different whole grains and combinations to create a variety of wholesome and delightful breakfast options for you and your family.

2. Fruit-Filled Delights: Sweet and Nutritious Breakfast Treats

Fruits are a delightful addition to breakfast, offering natural sweetness, essential vitamins, and antioxidants.

Here are some creative ways to prepare fruit-filled breakfast delights:

- Smoothie Bowls:
Blend a combination of your favorite fruits like bananas, berries, and mangoes with Greek yogurt or almond milk until smooth.
Pour the smoothie into a bowl and top with sliced fruits, granola, chia seeds, and a drizzle of honey for added texture and flavor.

- Fresh Fruit Salad:
Combine an assortment of seasonal fruits, such as strawberries, oranges, kiwi, and grapes, in a bowl.
Add a squeeze of fresh lemon juice and a sprinkle of mint leaves for a refreshing and vibrant fruit salad.

- Baked Apples:
Core apples and fill them with a mixture of chopped nuts, raisins, and cinnamon.
Bake until tender and serve warm with a dollop of Greek yogurt or a sprinkle of oats.

- Stuffed Berries:

Scoop out the center of strawberries or blueberries and fill them with a mixture of cream cheese and honey.
Chill before serving for a delightful and bite-sized treat.

- Fruit-Stuffed Crepes:
Prepare whole-grain crepes and fill them with sliced bananas, mixed berries, and a drizzle of pure maple syrup.
Fold the crepes and serve as a delicious and light breakfast.

- Tropical Fruit Parfait:
Layer diced mangoes, pineapple, and kiwi with coconut-flavored yogurt and toasted coconut flakes.
Repeat the layers and top with a few pieces of star fruit for a tropical-inspired parfait.

- Berry Compote:
Simmer mixed berries with a splash of water and a hint of honey until they release their juices and form a thick compote.
Serve over whole-grain toast or pancakes for a burst of natural sweetness.

These fruit-filled delights not only satisfy your sweet cravings but also provide essential nutrients, fiber, and antioxidants to kickstart your day on a healthy note.

Experiment with various fruit combinations to create a colorful and nutritious breakfast that will brighten your mornings and nourish your body.

3. Protein-Packed Options: Wholesome and Satisfying Breakfast Choices

Protein is an essential macronutrient that provides sustained energy, promotes satiety, and supports muscle repair and growth.

Here are some delicious and protein-packed breakfast options to fuel your morning:

- Veggie Omelet:

Whisk 2-3 eggs with a splash of milk.

Pour the mixture into a heated non-stick pan and add sautéed vegetables such as spinach, bell peppers, and tomatoes.

Sprinkle feta or goat cheese on top and fold the omelet in half.

- Greek Yogurt Parfait:

Layer Greek yogurt with a mix of fresh berries, sliced bananas, and a handful of granola.

Repeat the layers and top with a drizzle of honey or a sprinkle of chia seeds.

- Breakfast Burrito:

Fill a whole-grain tortilla with scrambled eggs, black beans, avocado slices, and salsa.

Roll it up and enjoy a savory and protein-rich handheld breakfast.

- Nut Butter Toast:

Spread natural almond or peanut butter on whole-grain toast.

Top with sliced bananas or strawberries and a sprinkle of chia seeds for added crunch and nutrition.

- Quinoa Breakfast Bowl:

Cook quinoa in water or milk according to package instructions.

Mix in a spoonful of honey, a handful of mixed nuts, and chopped dried fruits for a hearty and protein-packed bowl.

- Cottage Cheese Pancakes:

Combine cottage cheese, eggs, whole wheat flour, and a pinch of baking powder to create a pancake batter.
Cook spoonfuls of the batter on a non-stick pan and serve with fresh fruit and a dollop of yogurt.

- Protein Smoothie:
Blend a mix of frozen fruits, such as bananas, berries, and peaches, with your choice of protein powder and almond milk until smooth.
Add spinach or kale for extra nutrients and enjoy a nutrient-rich smoothie.

These protein-packed options not only provide essential amino acids but also support muscle health, satiety, and energy levels throughout the morning.
Customize these breakfast choices to your taste preferences and dietary needs, ensuring a nourishing and satisfying start to your day.

A. Mindful Portion Control: A Key to Healthy Eating and Blood Sugar Management

Mindful portion control involves paying close attention to the quantity of food consumed during meals and snacks. It is an essential practice for maintaining a balanced diet, managing blood sugar levels, and preventing overeating.

Here are some strategies for practicing mindful portion control:

1. Use Smaller Plates: Opt for smaller plates and bowls to create the illusion of a fuller plate, leading to satisfaction with smaller portions.

2. Listen to Hunger Cues: Pay attention to your body's hunger and fullness signals. Eat slowly, savoring each bite, and stop eating when you feel comfortably satisfied, not overly full.

3. Pre-Portion Snacks: Instead of eating directly from the package, portion snacks into small containers or bags to avoid mindlessly consuming large quantities.

4. Mindful Eating: Focus on the flavors, textures, and aromas of the food you are eating. Avoid distractions like TV or phones during mealtime to stay present and aware of your food intake.

5. Practice Balanced Meals: Aim to include a variety of nutrient-rich ingredients in each meal, such as whole grains, lean proteins, healthy fats, and plenty of fruits and vegetables.

6. Be Mindful of Liquid Calories: Pay attention to beverage choices, as liquid calories from sugary drinks can quickly add up. Opt for water, herbal tea, or unsweetened beverages whenever possible.

7. Avoid Emotional Eating: Be mindful of eating habits triggered by emotions, stress, or boredom. Seek alternative coping mechanisms such as exercise or meditation.

8. Plan Ahead: Plan meals and snacks in advance to avoid impulse eating and ensure balanced and appropriate portion sizes.

By practicing mindful portion control, individuals can enjoy their meals, maintain healthy blood sugar levels, and prevent weight gain or other health concerns related to excessive caloric intake.
Being mindful of portion sizes fosters a healthier relationship with food and supports overall well-being.

Collaborating with healthcare providers is a crucial aspect of managing diabetes and kidney health effectively. Healthcare providers, including doctors, nurses, dietitians, and diabetes educators, play a vital role in developing personalized treatment plans, monitoring health progress, and providing essential support throughout the journey.

Here's why collaborating with healthcare providers is essential:

1. Personalized Care: Healthcare providers tailor treatment plans based on individual health needs, medical history, and lifestyle preferences. This personalized approach ensures the most effective management of diabetes and kidney health.

2. Monitoring Health Parameters: Healthcare providers regularly monitor blood sugar levels, kidney function, blood pressure, and other vital health parameters. These measurements provide valuable insights into the effectiveness of the treatment plan and aid in making necessary adjustments.

3. Medication Management: Healthcare providers prescribe and manage medications for diabetes and kidney health, adjusting dosages or introducing new therapies as needed to achieve optimal health outcomes.

4. Nutritional Guidance: Dietitians collaborate with patients to develop balanced meal plans, incorporating nutrient-rich ingredients and considering specific dietary restrictions related to diabetes and kidney health.

5. Lifestyle Modifications: Healthcare providers offer guidance on lifestyle modifications, including regular physical activity, stress management, and smoking cessation, which significantly impact diabetes and kidney health.

6. Education and Support: Diabetes educators and healthcare providers offer valuable education and support, empowering individuals to understand their conditions better and take an active role in their health management.

7. Preventive Care: Regular check-ups and screenings with healthcare providers allow for early detection of potential complications, enabling timely intervention to prevent further health issues.

Collaborating with healthcare providers fosters a team-based approach to managing diabetes and kidney health. By actively participating in treatment decisions and following their guidance, individuals can achieve better health outcomes, improve their quality of life, and reduce the risk of diabetes-related complications.
Regular communication with healthcare providers ensures ongoing support and adjustments to treatment plans as needed, leading to better long-term health management.

In Summary
A wholesome and delightful breakfast sets the tone for a successful day, particularly for individuals with diabetes.
By incorporating nutrient-rich ingredients, practising portion control, and collaborating with healthcare providers, individuals can enjoy breakfast delights that promote blood sugar control, support overall health, and contribute to improved diabetes management.

Starting the day with nourishing breakfast choices ensures a positive impact on blood glucose levels and enhances overall well-being for individuals with diabetes.

Chapter Five

Satisfying Lunches: A Blend of Taste and Health

Lunch is an important meal that fuels us with energy and nutrients to carry through the day. When it comes to crafting satisfying lunches, finding the perfect balance between taste and health is essential. A well-balanced lunch should be delicious, filling, and packed with nutrient-rich ingredients that support overall well-being. In this comprehensive guide, we will explore various satisfying lunch options that cater to different tastes, dietary preferences, and health needs.

The Importance of a Balanced Lunch

A balanced lunch is an essential part of a healthy and productive day. It provides the body with the necessary nutrients and energy to sustain physical and mental activities, maintain blood sugar levels, and support overall well-being.

Here are some reasons why a balanced lunch is crucial:

I. Sustained Energy: A balanced lunch includes a mix of carbohydrates, proteins, and healthy fats, which provide sustained energy throughout the afternoon. Carbohydrates break down into glucose, providing immediate energy, while proteins and fats offer longer-lasting energy.

II. Improved Focus and Concentration: Proper nutrition at lunchtime enhances cognitive function and concentration. Nutrient-rich foods support brain health and cognitive processes, leading to increased productivity and better performance.

III. Blood Sugar Management: Balancing carbohydrates with proteins and fats helps regulate blood sugar levels. This prevents rapid spikes and crashes in blood glucose, reducing the risk of energy slumps and mood fluctuations.

IV. Weight Management: A balanced lunch with appropriate portion sizes prevents overeating later in the day. Including fiber-rich foods like fruits, vegetables, and whole grains promotes feelings of fullness and aids in weight management.

V. Supporting Nutrient Intake: Lunch provides an opportunity to include nutrient-rich ingredients such as vegetables, fruits, lean proteins, and whole grains, which contribute to essential vitamins, minerals, and antioxidants.

VI. Digestive Health: A well-balanced lunch with a mix of fiber, proteins, and fats supports healthy digestion and prevents issues like bloating and discomfort.

VII. Preventing Unhealthy Snacking: A satisfying lunch reduces the likelihood of reaching for unhealthy snacks later in the day, promoting better food choices and supporting long-term health goals.

VIII. Muscle Repair and Maintenance: Proteins in a balanced lunch are essential for muscle repair and maintenance, making it crucial for individuals engaged in physical activity or exercise.

IX. Immune Support: Nutrient-rich lunches provide the body with the necessary components to support the immune system, reducing the risk of illness and infections.

X. Positive Impact on Overall Health: Consistently consuming balanced lunches contributes to better overall health, reducing the risk of chronic diseases such as diabetes, cardiovascular issues, and obesity.

By prioritizing a balanced lunch, individuals can optimize their daily performance, support overall health, and cultivate healthy eating habits. A well-balanced midday meal ensures that the body receives the necessary nutrients and energy to tackle the day's challenges with vitality and focus.

1. Nutrient-Rich Ingredients for Lunch:
Incorporating nutrient-rich ingredients into lunch options is a great way to boost the nutritional value of the midday meal.
These ingredients are packed with essential vitamins, minerals, antioxidants, and other beneficial compounds that support overall health and well-being.

Here are some nutrient-rich ingredients to include in your lunch:

- **Leafy Greens:** Spinach, kale, arugula, and Swiss chard are excellent sources of vitamins A, C, K, and various minerals like iron and calcium.
- **Colorful Vegetables:** Bell peppers, carrots, tomatoes, cucumbers, and broccoli provide a wide range of vitamins, antioxidants, and dietary fiber.

- **Lean Proteins:** Grilled chicken, turkey, tofu, tempeh, beans, lentils, and quinoa are excellent sources of protein, essential for muscle repair and overall health.

- **Whole Grains:** Brown rice, quinoa, barley, farro, and whole wheat bread offer complex carbohydrates, fiber, and essential nutrients.

- **Healthy Fats:** Avocado, nuts, seeds, and olive oil provide healthy monounsaturated and polyunsaturated fats, beneficial for heart health and nutrient absorption.

- **Berries:** Blueberries, strawberries, raspberries, and blackberries are rich in antioxidants, vitamin C, and dietary fiber.

- **Citrus Fruits:** Oranges, grapefruits, and lemons are high in vitamin C and other antioxidants, supporting the immune system.

- **Cruciferous Vegetables:** Broccoli, cauliflower, and Brussels sprouts offer unique compounds that have been linked to cancer prevention and overall health.

- **Fatty Fish:** Salmon, mackerel, and sardines are rich in omega-3 fatty acids, supporting heart and brain health.

- **Greek Yogurt:** A good source of protein and probiotics, promoting gut health and supporting digestion.
- **Legumes:** Chickpeas, lentils, and beans are rich sources of fibre, protein, and a number of vitamins and minerals.
- **Sweet Potatoes:** Rich in vitamin A, C, and potassium, sweet potatoes provide a nutrient-dense carbohydrate option.
- **Herbs and Spices:** Fresh herbs like basil, cilantro, and mint, as well as spices like turmeric, ginger, and cinnamon, add flavor and provide additional health benefits.

Including a variety of these nutrient-rich ingredients in your lunch helps ensure you get a diverse range of essential nutrients, promoting overall health and well-being. You can combine these ingredients creatively to create salads, wraps, bowls, soups, and other satisfying and nutrient-packed lunch options.

2. Mindful Portion Control at Lunch:

Mindful portion control at lunch involves being present and conscious of the food choices and quantities consumed during the midday meal. It is a practice that encourages eating in moderation, fostering a balanced and healthy diet.

By paying attention to hunger cues, serving sizes, and nutritional needs, mindful portion control supports overall well-being, weight management, and optimal nutrition.

Here are some practical tips for practicing mindful portion control at lunch:

I. Gauge Your Hunger: Before eating, take a moment to assess your hunger level. Are you genuinely hungry, or are you eating out of habit or emotions? Mindful eating starts with understanding your body's true hunger signals.

II. Use Smaller Plates or Containers: Opt for smaller lunch plates or containers to encourage smaller portions. This helps prevent overeating and promotes the feeling of satisfaction with less food.

III. Prioritize Nutrient-Rich Foods: Center your lunch around nutrient-dense ingredients like vegetables, fruits, lean proteins, and whole grains. To support general health, these foods offer necessary vitamins, minerals, and antioxidants.

IV. Be Mindful of Serving Sizes: Pay attention to serving sizes for different food groups. Aim for a balanced plate with appropriate portions of proteins, carbohydrates, and vegetables.

V. Slow Down and Savor: Eat your lunch slowly, savoring each bite. Chew thoroughly and take time to appreciate the flavors and textures of your meal. Mindful eating allows you to enjoy your food fully and recognize when you're satisfied.

VI. Mindful Snacking: If you include snacks with your lunch, portion them mindfully in separate containers. Avoid eating directly from a large bag or container to prevent mindless overeating.

VII. Stay Hydrated: Drink water throughout your meal, as proper hydration can help control appetite and prevent overeating.

VIII. Reduce Distractions: Avoid engaging in activities like TV watching or phone scrolling while you are eating. Focus solely on your meal to avoid mindless consumption.

IX. Tune into Fullness: Pause halfway through your meal and check in with your body to assess how full you feel. If you are satisfied, consider saving the rest for later or a subsequent meal.

X. Plan Your Lunches: Plan your lunches in advance, incorporating a variety of nutrient-rich ingredients. Meal preparation allows you to control portion sizes and make healthier choices.

XI. Embrace Flexibility: Be flexible with your lunch choices and enjoy a diverse range of foods. Avoid strict rules or restrictions that may lead to feelings of deprivation.

Practicing mindful portion control at lunch fosters a positive relationship with food, promotes better digestion, and supports weight management goals.
By being aware of your body's needs and making intentional food choices, you can nourish yourself with balance and make lunchtime a satisfying and healthful experience.

3. Protein-Packed Lunch Ideas: Satisfying and Nourishing Midday Meals

Including protein in your lunch is essential for maintaining energy levels, supporting muscle repair, and promoting overall health.
Protein-rich lunches provide satiety and help prevent the urge to snack between meals.

Here are some delicious and protein-packed lunch ideas to keep you fueled and satisfied throughout the day:

- Grilled Chicken Salad:

Create a refreshing salad with grilled chicken breast, mixed greens, cherry tomatoes, cucumbers, avocado slices, and a sprinkle of feta cheese.

Dress it with a lemon vinaigrette for added flavor.

- Quinoa Buddha Bowl:

Prepare a nutrient-dense bowl with cooked quinoa, roasted chickpeas, sautéed spinach, cherry tomatoes, shredded carrots, and sliced avocado.

Top it off with a tahini dressing for a creamy finish.

- Turkey and Hummus Wrap:

Spread hummus on a whole wheat wrap and layer it with sliced turkey, lettuce, tomatoes, cucumbers, and shredded carrots.

Roll it up for a quick and satisfying handheld lunch.

- Tofu Stir-Fry:

Toss cubed tofu with mixed vegetables like bell peppers, broccoli, and snap peas in a flavorful stir-fry sauce.

Serve it over brown rice or quinoa for a plant-based protein-packed meal.

- Lentil Soup:

Prepare a hearty lentil soup with red or green lentils, carrots, celery, onions, and vegetable broth.

Add a touch of spices like cumin and coriander for a comforting and protein-rich lunch option.

- Chickpea Salad:

Combine chickpeas with chopped cucumbers, red onions, cherry tomatoes, and fresh parsley.

Dress the salad with a lemon and olive oil dressing for a light and protein-packed lunch.

- Salmon Quinoa Bowl:

Cook quinoa and top it with baked or grilled salmon, steamed asparagus, and a drizzle of lemon-dill sauce.

This bowl provides a healthy dose of omega-3 fatty acids and protein.

- Egg Salad Lettuce Wraps:

Mix hard-boiled eggs with Greek yogurt, Dijon mustard, celery, and green onions.

Serve the egg salad in lettuce wraps for a light and protein-filled lunch.

- Black Bean Burrito Bowl:

Create a burrito bowl with black beans, brown rice, sautéed bell peppers, onions, and corn.

Top it with avocado slices and a dollop of Greek yogurt for added creaminess.

- Chicken Avocado Salad:

Combine cooked chicken breast with diced avocado, cherry tomatoes, red onions, and cilantro.

Season it with lime juice, salt, and pepper for a refreshing and protein-rich salad.

These protein-packed lunch ideas cater to various dietary preferences and are easy to prepare for busy weekdays. Including a variety of protein sources in your lunch ensures that you get the necessary nutrients to support your active lifestyle and overall well-being.

4. Vegetarian and Vegan Lunches: Delicious and Nutritious Plant-Based Options

Vegetarian and vegan lunches offer a wide array of flavorful and nutrient-dense options that cater to plant-based dietary preferences.

These lunches are not only delicious but also packed with essential vitamins, minerals, and plant-based proteins.

Whether you follow a vegetarian or vegan lifestyle or simply want to incorporate more plant-based meals into your diet,

Here are some satisfying lunch ideas:

- Vegan Buddha Bowl:

Create a colorful bowl with a base of quinoa or brown rice, topped with roasted vegetables like sweet potatoes, Brussels sprouts, and broccoli.
Add chickpeas or black beans for protein, and drizzle with tahini or avocado dressing.

- Caprese Avocado Salad:
Layer sliced avocados with juicy tomatoes, fresh basil leaves, and vegan mozzarella or tofu.
Drizzle with balsamic glaze and olive oil for a refreshing and filling salad.

- Vegetable Stir-Fry:
Sauté an assortment of colorful vegetables like bell peppers, zucchini, carrots, and snow peas in a savory vegan stir-fry sauce.
Serve it over noodles or quinoa for a satisfying lunch.

- Vegan Chickpea Tuna Salad:
Mash chickpeas with vegan mayo, Dijon mustard, chopped celery, and red onions to create a plant-based tuna salad.
Enjoy it in a sandwich or lettuce wrap.

- Lentil and Vegetable Curry:

Prepare a flavorful lentil curry with an assortment of vegetables like cauliflower, carrots, and bell peppers.
Serve it over brown rice or quinoa for a protein-rich lunch.

- Vegan Mediterranean Wrap:
Fill a whole wheat wrap with hummus, sliced cucumbers, cherry tomatoes, olives, and fresh greens.
Add a sprinkle of vegan feta cheese for a Mediterranean-inspired lunch.

- Vegan Sushi Bowl:
Create a deconstructed sushi bowl with sushi rice, avocado slices, cucumber, and pickled ginger.
Add marinated tofu or edamame for a protein boost.

- Vegan Black Bean Quesadilla:
Stuff a whole wheat tortilla with mashed black beans, vegan cheese, diced bell peppers, and onions.
Cook until crispy and serve with guacamole or salsa.

- Vegan Cauliflower Buffalo Wings:
Bread cauliflower florets with a mixture of flour and plant-based milk, then bake until crispy.

Toss them in buffalo sauce for a spicy and satisfying lunch.

- Vegan Lentil Shepherd's Pie:
Layer cooked lentils, mixed vegetables, and mashed sweet potatoes or cauliflower in a casserole dish.
Bake until golden and enjoy a comforting and nutritious lunch.

These vegetarian and vegan lunch ideas showcase the versatility and creativity of plant-based cooking. Whether you're looking for a light and refreshing salad or a hearty and filling bowl, there are numerous options to suit your taste preferences and dietary needs.
Embracing plant-based lunches not only promotes health and well-being but also benefits the environment and supports sustainable food choices.

5. Gluten-Free Lunch Options: Tasty and Wholesome Choices for Gluten Sensitivity
For individuals with gluten sensitivity or celiac disease, finding satisfying gluten-free lunch options is essential to maintain a balanced and enjoyable diet. Fortunately, there are numerous delicious and

wholesome gluten-free lunch ideas that cater to various tastes and dietary preferences.

Here are some tasty gluten-free lunch options to explore:

- Quinoa Salad:
Prepare a refreshing quinoa salad with a mix of colorful vegetables, such as cherry tomatoes, cucumber, bell peppers, and red onion.
Add fresh herbs like parsley or cilantro and dress it with a lemon vinaigrette.

- Rice Paper Rolls:
Fill rice paper wraps with rice noodles, avocado slices, shredded carrots, cucumber, lettuce, and fresh herbs.
Dip them in a gluten-free peanut sauce for a light and flavorful lunch.

- Gluten-Free Wraps:
Opt for gluten-free wraps made from corn, rice, or other alternative flours.
Fill them with grilled chicken, hummus, roasted vegetables, and leafy greens.

- Zucchini Noodles:
Create "zoodles" with spiralized zucchini and toss them with gluten-free marinara sauce and vegan meatballs or cooked shrimp.

- Stuffed Bell Peppers:
Fill halved bell peppers with a mix of cooked quinoa, black beans, corn, and diced tomatoes.
Top them with dairy-free cheese and bake until tender.

- Lentil Salad:
Make a hearty lentil salad with cooked lentils, diced celery, red bell pepper, and green onions.
Dress it with a tangy vinaigrette for added flavor.

- Sushi Bowls:
Prepare a sushi-inspired bowl with sushi rice, sliced avocado, cucumber, pickled ginger, and your favorite protein like cooked shrimp or tofu.

- Baked Sweet Potatoes:
Top baked sweet potatoes with black beans, avocado slices, and a sprinkle of dairy-free cheese or nutritional yeast.

- Quiche Cups:
Create gluten-free quiche cups using a combination of eggs, dairy-free milk, and assorted vegetables.
Bake them in muffin tins for easy portioning.

- Stir-Fry with Tamari Sauce:
Stir-fry a mix of colorful vegetables with your choice of protein like chicken, tofu, or tempeh.
Use gluten-free tamari sauce for a savory flavor.

- Chicken Lettuce Wraps:
Replace the traditional wrap with lettuce leaves and fill them with seasoned ground chicken, water chestnuts, and diced vegetables.

- Gazpacho:
Enjoy a refreshing cold gazpacho soup made with ripe tomatoes, cucumbers, bell peppers, and fresh herbs.

When preparing gluten-free lunches, always check labels and ingredients to ensure they are free of gluten.
Additionally, opt for whole, unprocessed foods whenever possible to support a balanced and nutritious diet.

With creativity and attention to gluten-free ingredients, you can savor a wide range of delicious and safe lunch options that cater to your dietary needs.

6. Make-Ahead Lunches for Convenience: Enjoy Delicious Meals with Minimal Effort

Make-ahead lunches are a time-saving and convenient solution for busy individuals looking to enjoy delicious and nourishing meals throughout the week. By preparing lunches in advance, you can avoid the last-minute scramble and ensure that you have satisfying options readily available.

Here are some make-ahead lunch ideas to simplify your daily routine:

- Mason Jar Salads:
Layer your favorite salad ingredients in mason jars, starting with dressing at the bottom, followed by sturdy vegetables, proteins, and leafy greens on top.
Refrigerate the jars with their lids on until you're ready to eat.
Shake the jar before enjoying your fresh and crisp salad.

- Prepped Grains and Proteins:

Cook a batch of quinoa, brown rice, or roasted sweet potatoes and store them in separate containers.

Prepare protein options like grilled chicken, marinated tofu, or boiled eggs.

Combine them with fresh vegetables or toss them into salads for quick and easy lunches.

- Freezer-Friendly Soups and Stews:

Make large batches of hearty soups or stews and freeze individual portions in resealable bags or containers.

Just thaw and reheat for a comforting and satisfying lunch.

- DIY Lunchables:

Create your own healthier version of lunchables by packing whole grain crackers, sliced cheese, hummus, and a variety of colorful fruits and vegetables in a bento-style container.

- Veggie Wraps:

Prepare wraps or burritos with your favorite fillings like hummus, avocado, roasted vegetables, and beans.

Roll them up, wrap them in foil, and store them in the fridge for a convenient grab-and-go lunch.

- Overnight Oats:

Combine rolled oats, plant-based milk, chia seeds, and your favorite toppings in a jar.

Let it sit in the fridge overnight, and you'll have a delicious and nutritious breakfast or lunch option.

- Mason Jar Noodles:

Layer cooked rice noodles or soba noodles, vegetables, and protein with a flavorful sauce in mason jars.

Add boiling water at lunchtime and let it sit for a few minutes before enjoying a hot noodle meal.

- Baked Casseroles:

Prepare casseroles with your choice of vegetables, proteins, and sauces.

Bake them in a large dish and portion them into individual containers for easy reheating.

- DIY Salad Kits:

Create individual salad kits by placing washed and chopped salad ingredients in separate containers.

Assemble your salad quickly by combining the components at lunchtime.

- Energy Bites or Bars:
Make a batch of homemade energy bites or granola bars for a quick and satisfying snack to accompany your lunch.

Make-ahead lunches not only save time but also ensure that you're nourished with balanced and wholesome meals.
Set aside some time on the weekend or during the week to prepare these meals, and you'll have the convenience of enjoying delicious homemade lunches without the hassle of cooking each day.

7. Leftovers Reinvented: Transforming Yesterday's Meals into Today's Delights

Leftovers can be a treasure trove of ingredients to create exciting and innovative meals. By reinventing leftovers, you can save time, reduce food waste, and enjoy a variety of delicious dishes without feeling like you're eating the same thing repeatedly.

Here are some creative ways to breathe new life into your leftovers:

- Turn Stir-Fry into Fried Rice:
Use leftover stir-fry vegetables, proteins, and rice to make a flavorful fried rice.
Simply sauté the ingredients in a pan with some soy sauce and other seasonings of your choice.

- Repurpose Roasted Vegetables:
Roasted vegetables can be used in a multitude of dishes.
Add them to omelets, pasta dishes, salads, or even sandwiches for an extra burst of flavor and nutrients.

- Remix Salad Ingredients:
Use leftover salad components to create unique grain bowls or wraps.
Combine greens, protein, and toppings with cooked quinoa, couscous, or your favorite grain.

- Create Buddha Bowls:
Combine various leftovers like grains, roasted vegetables, cooked beans, and protein to create colorful and nutritious Buddha bowls.

- Make Breakfast Hash:

Transform leftover roasted potatoes, vegetables, and proteins into a hearty breakfast hash.
Add some eggs for a complete morning meal.

- Reinvent Pasta Dishes:
Turn pasta leftovers into a pasta bake by layering them with cheese and tomato sauce.
Bake until golden and bubbly for a comforting meal.

- Transform Soups into Sauces:
Use leftover soup as a flavorful sauce for pasta or rice dishes.
Blend the soup to make it smooth or use it as is for added texture.

- Stuff Veggies with Grains and Proteins:
Stuff bell peppers, zucchinis, or tomatoes with leftover grains and proteins.
For a nice and nutritious lunch, bake the food until it is soft.

- Reinvent Tacos:
Use leftover taco fillings to create delicious quesadillas or taco salads.
Simply add cheese between tortillas and cook until melted, or toss the toppings with salad greens.

- Reimagine Pizza Toppings:

Transform pizza toppings into a frittata or omelet for a breakfast or brunch option.

- Make Sushi Rolls:

Use leftover grains, vegetables, and proteins to make sushi rolls or sushi bowls.

These reinvented rolls are great for a light and refreshing lunch.

- Reinvent Desserts:

Turn leftover fruit into smoothies, compotes, or fruit crisps.

Use stale bread for bread pudding or French toast.

By thinking creatively and repurposing leftovers, you can add variety and excitement to your meals while reducing food waste.

Experiment with different combinations, flavors, and cooking methods to reinvent your leftovers into enjoyable and satisfying dishes. With a little imagination, yesterday's meals can become today's culinary delights.

8. Incorporating Superfoods: Elevating Nutrition and Flavor in Your Diet

Superfoods are nutrient-dense foods that are rich in vitamins, minerals, antioxidants, and other beneficial compounds. By incorporating these powerhouse ingredients into your diet, you can boost your overall nutrition and support your well-being.

Here are some tips on how to include superfoods in your daily meals:

I. Berries: Add a handful of blueberries, strawberries, or raspberries to your breakfast smoothie, oatmeal, or yogurt. Berries are packed with antioxidants and provide a natural sweetness to your meals.

II. Leafy Greens: Enjoy a variety of leafy greens like spinach, kale, or Swiss chard in salads, wraps, or sautés. Excellent sources of vitamins and minerals can be found in these greens.

III. Avocado: Spread avocado on toast, add it to salads, or use it as a creamy base for dressings and sauces. Avocado is rich in healthy fats and provides a creamy texture to your dishes.

IV. Nuts and Seeds: Sprinkle chia seeds, flaxseeds, or hemp seeds over your smoothies, salads, or yogurt for an extra boost of omega-3 fatty acids and fiber.

V. Quinoa: Swap traditional grains with quinoa in salads, stir-fries, or as a side dish. Quinoa has all nine essential amino acids and is a complete protein.

VI. Beans and Legumes: Incorporate black beans, chickpeas, or lentils into soups, stews, and salads. These plant-based proteins are rich in fiber and help stabilize blood sugar levels.

VII. Turmeric: Add a pinch of turmeric to curries, rice dishes, or smoothies. Turmeric contains curcumin, a potent anti-inflammatory compound.

VIII. Sweet Potatoes: Roast or bake sweet potatoes and enjoy them as a side dish or use them as a base for bowls and salads. Sweet potatoes are a good source of vitamins and antioxidants.

IX. Greek Yogurt: Opt for Greek yogurt, which is high in protein, calcium, and probiotics. Use it as a creamy topping for fruits or in place of sour cream in recipes.

X. Dark Chocolate: Enjoy a small piece of dark chocolate with a high cocoa content as a satisfying and antioxidant-rich treat.

XI. Seaweed: Incorporate seaweed, such as nori or dulse, into homemade sushi rolls, salads, or soups. Seaweed is rich in iodine and other trace minerals.

XII. Matcha: Use matcha powder in smoothies, lattes, or baked goods for an energy-boosting and antioxidant-packed addition.

When incorporating superfoods into your meals, remember to balance them with a variety of other nutritious foods to achieve a well-rounded diet.

Watch your portion sizes and pay attention to your body's hunger signals. By making superfoods a regular part of your meals, you can enhance your nutrition and overall health while enjoying a delicious and vibrant culinary experience.

9. Hydration and Beverages: Nourishing Your Body with Healthy Fluids

Staying hydrated is crucial for overall well-being and optimal bodily functions. Water is essential for regulating body temperature, aiding digestion, transporting nutrients, and flushing out waste.

In addition to plain water, various beverages can contribute to hydration and provide additional health benefits.

Here's a guide to hydration and beverage choices:

I. Water: Water should be your go-to beverage for hydration. Aim to drink at least 8 cups (64 ounces) of water per day, but individual needs may vary based on factors like age, activity level, and climate.

II. Herbal Teas: Herbal teas, like chamomile, peppermint, or rooibos, are caffeine-free options that offer a comforting and hydrating alternative. Many herbal teas also contain antioxidants and may have calming effects.

III. Green Tea: Green tea is a low-calorie beverage that contains antioxidants and may help boost metabolism and support cardiovascular health. Enjoy it hot or cold without added sugar or sweeteners.

IV. Infused Water: Enhance the flavor of water by infusing it with fresh fruits, herbs, or cucumber slices. This adds a refreshing taste without any added sugars.

V. Coconut Water: Coconut water is a natural source of electrolytes, making it a great option for rehydration after exercise or exposure to heat.

VI. Fresh Fruit Juices: While whole fruits are preferred for their fiber content, occasional consumption of fresh fruit juices can provide vitamins and minerals. Opt for 100% natural fruit juices without added sugars.

VII. Nut Milks: Nut milks like almond, cashew, or oat milk can be used as a dairy-free alternative and are often fortified with essential nutrients like calcium and vitamin D.

VIII. Smoothies: Wholesome smoothies made with fruits, vegetables, and plant-based milk can be hydrating and nutrient-dense. Avoid adding excessive sugars or syrups.

IX. Kombucha: Kombucha is a fermented beverage rich in probiotics, which can support gut health. Choose low-sugar varieties for a hydrating and refreshing option.

X. Lemon Water: Add a squeeze of fresh lemon or lime to your water for a touch of flavor and extra vitamin C.

While incorporating various beverages into your diet, be mindful of added sugars, artificial sweeteners, and excessive caffeine consumption. Water should remain the primary source of hydration, and other beverages can complement your fluid intake while providing additional health benefits.

Balancing hydration with a diverse range of healthy beverages can contribute to a well-hydrated and nourished body.

10. Mindful Eating Habits:

Practicing mindful eating during lunch encourages enjoying each bite, savoring flavors, and being present. Minimizing distractions and focusing on the meal fosters a more satisfying dining experience.

11. Collaborating with Healthcare Providers:

Individuals with specific health conditions or dietary restrictions can benefit from collaborating with healthcare providers and registered dietitians to tailor lunch choices that align with their health goals.

In Summary

Crafting satisfying lunches that balance taste and health is a fulfilling and enjoyable endeavor. By incorporating nutrient-rich ingredients, mindful portion control, and creative combinations, individuals can create lunch options that nourish the body, support energy levels, and contribute to overall well-being.

Embracing a variety of tastes, textures, and cuisines in lunch choices ensures a satisfying and nutritious midday meal experience. By making lunchtime a priority for nourishing the body and mind, individuals can reap the benefits of improved health, productivity, and overall satisfaction in their daily lives.

Chapter Six

Delectable Dinners for Diabetic Renal Diets: Nourishing Meals for Healthy Kidneys

A diabetic renal diet is a specialized eating plan designed to support both diabetes management and kidney health. For individuals with diabetes and chronic kidney disease (CKD), maintaining a balanced diet is crucial to prevent further kidney damage and manage blood sugar levels effectively. By focusing on nutrient-dense and kidney-friendly ingredients, delectable dinners can be created that cater to both dietary restrictions and delicious flavors. In this comprehensive guide, we will explore various aspects of delectable dinners for diabetic renal diets, including the principles of a renal-friendly diet, essential nutrients, and a diverse selection of kidney-friendly dinner recipes.

Principles of a Diabetic Renal Diet

The principles of a diabetic renal diet are a set of dietary guidelines designed to address the specific nutritional needs of individuals living with both diabetes and chronic kidney disease (CKD). This specialized eating plan aims to promote kidney health, manage blood sugar levels, and prevent further kidney damage. By following these principles, individuals can make informed food choices that cater to their unique medical conditions and support their overall well-being.

1. Limiting Sodium: Reducing sodium intake is essential to manage blood pressure and fluid balance. Sodium-rich ingredients like processed foods, canned goods, and condiments should be avoided or limited.

2. Moderating Protein Intake: For individuals with kidney disease, controlling protein intake helps alleviate the strain on the kidneys. Consuming high-quality protein sources in appropriate portions is essential.

3. Monitoring Potassium and Phosphorus: As kidneys may struggle to filter these minerals, it's important to be mindful of potassium and phosphorus levels in the diet. Choosing low-potassium and low-phosphorus foods can help maintain kidney function.

4. Managing Carbohydrates: For individuals with diabetes, controlling carbohydrate intake is crucial to manage blood sugar levels. Choosing complex carbohydrates and monitoring portion sizes is key.

5. Adequate Fluid Intake: Ensuring sufficient fluid intake is necessary for kidney health. However, individuals with advanced CKD may need to limit fluid intake to prevent fluid retention.

6. Balancing Nutrients: Designing meals that strike the right balance of nutrients, including carbohydrates, protein, fats, vitamins, and minerals, is essential for overall health and well-being.

Essential Nutrients for Diabetic Renal Diets: Vital Components for Kidney Health and Diabetes Management

Essential nutrients for diabetic renal diets are the key components necessary to support kidney health and effectively manage diabetes while meeting the unique nutritional needs of individuals with both conditions. These nutrients play a crucial role in promoting overall well-being, blood sugar control, and maintaining optimal kidney function. By incorporating these essential nutrients into their diets, individuals can ensure that their nutritional intake aligns with their medical conditions, supporting both diabetes management and kidney health.

1. Low-Potassium Vegetables: Incorporate kidney-friendly vegetables like bell peppers, cauliflower, cabbage, green beans, and lettuce.

2. Low-Phosphorus Proteins: Opt for lean proteins with lower phosphorus content, such as poultry, fish, eggs, and tofu.

3. Healthy Fats: Include sources of healthy fats like avocados, olive oil, nuts, and seeds for heart health.

4. High-Fiber Foods: Fiber-rich foods like whole grains, legumes, and vegetables can help manage blood sugar levels and promote digestive health.

5. Diabetic-Friendly Fruits: Choose fruits that are lower in sugar and potassium, such as berries, apples, and cherries.

Delicious Dinner Recipes for Diabetic Renal Diets

- Grilled Lemon Herb Chicken:
Combine lemon juice, garlic, and herbs in a marinade for chicken breasts.
Grill until tender and serve with steamed green beans and quinoa.

- Baked Salmon with Dill Sauce:
Season salmon fillets with dill, garlic, and a dash of lemon juice.
Bake until flaky and serve with a side of roasted asparagus.

- Turkey and Vegetable Stir-Fry:
Sauté lean ground turkey with a variety of colorful vegetables like bell peppers, broccoli, and snap peas.
Season with low-sodium soy sauce and ginger, and serve over cauliflower rice.

- Mediterranean Stuffed Bell Peppers:

Fill halved bell peppers with a mixture of cooked quinoa, black beans, tomatoes, and fresh herbs.
Bake until tender and top with crumbled feta cheese (in moderation).

- Eggplant Parmesan:
Layer thinly sliced eggplant with marinara sauce and mozzarella cheese (in moderation).
Bake until bubbly and serve with a side of mixed greens.

- Spinach and Feta Stuffed Chicken:
Stuff chicken breasts with a mixture of sautéed spinach and crumbled feta cheese (in moderation).
Bake until chicken is cooked through.

- Zucchini Noodles with Shrimp and Pesto:
Spiralize zucchini to create noodles and sauté with cooked shrimp and homemade pesto made from basil, garlic, pine nuts, and olive oil.

- Cauliflower and Broccoli Casserole:
Create a creamy casserole with cauliflower and broccoli florets, topped with a mixture of Greek yogurt and shredded cheese (in moderation).

- Lentil and Vegetable Curry:
Prepare a flavorful curry with lentils, tomatoes, and an array of kidney-friendly vegetables like carrots, green beans, and spinach.
Serve with brown rice.

- Quinoa-Stuffed Portobello Mushrooms:
Mix cooked quinoa with diced tomatoes, onions, and seasonings.
Stuff into portobello mushroom caps and bake until tender.

In Summary
These delectable dinner recipes for diabetic renal diets showcase the diverse and flavorful options available while adhering to the principles of a kidney-friendly and diabetes-friendly eating plan.
By focusing on nutrient-rich ingredients, controlling portion sizes, and practicing mindful eating habits, individuals can enjoy satisfying and nourishing meals that support both diabetes and kidney health.
Always consult with a healthcare provider or a registered dietitian before making significant changes to your diet, especially if you have specific medical conditions or dietary restrictions. With a thoughtful approach to meal planning and cooking,

individuals can embark on a culinary journey that nurtures their well-being and taste buds alike.

Chapter Seven

Nourishing Snacks for Energy and Satisfaction: A Guide to Healthy and Satisfying Choices

Snacking plays an essential role in maintaining energy levels, managing hunger, and providing essential nutrients between meals. Choosing nourishing snacks can support overall health, keep blood sugar levels stable, and provide a sense of satisfaction.

Whether you need a quick pick-me-up during a busy day or a post-workout refuel, selecting snacks that are balanced, nutrient-dense, and enjoyable can promote well-being and prevent unhealthy cravings.

In this comprehensive guide, we will explore the principles of nourishing snacking, the importance of balanced choices, and a variety of delicious snack ideas that cater to different dietary preferences and nutritional needs.

The principles of nourishing snacking are a set of guidelines that help individuals make mindful and healthful choices when selecting snacks. These principles aim to ensure that snacks are not just a source of quick energy but also provide a balance of essential nutrients to support overall health and well-being. By adhering to these principles, individuals can make nourishing snacking a part of their daily routine, promoting sustained energy, managing hunger, and preventing unhealthy cravings.

1. Balanced Macronutrients: Aim to include a combination of carbohydrates, proteins, and healthy fats in your snacks. This balance helps maintain steady blood sugar levels, provides sustained energy, and keeps you feeling full and satisfied.

2. Nutrient Density: Opt for snacks that offer a wealth of essential nutrients, such as vitamins, minerals, fiber, and antioxidants. This can be achieved by choosing whole foods like fruits, vegetables, nuts, and seeds.

3. Mindful Portion Control: Be mindful of portion sizes to avoid excessive calorie intake. Pre-portioning snacks or using small containers can help control portions and prevent overeating.

4. Minimize Added Sugars and Processed Foods: Limit snacks that are high in added sugars, refined carbohydrates, and unhealthy fats. Consider full, healthy foods that fuel your body instead.

5. Hydration: Remember to hydrate throughout the day, as proper hydration is essential for overall health and energy levels.

Importance of Balanced Snacks

Snacking is an integral part of our daily routine, providing us with the necessary energy to power through busy days and maintain focus between meals. However, not all snacks are created equal, and the choices we make can significantly impact our health and well-being. The importance of balanced snacks cannot be overstated, as they play a crucial role in keeping us nourished, energized, and satisfied throughout the day.

A balanced snack is one that combines essential nutrients, such as carbohydrates, proteins, and healthy fats, in the right proportions. This harmonious blend ensures that our blood sugar levels remain stable, preventing energy crashes and sudden hunger pangs. Beyond merely filling the gap between meals, balanced snacks provide a range of benefits that contribute to our overall health and vitality.

In this guide, we delve into the significance of incorporating balanced snacks into our daily lives. We explore how they help maintain steady energy levels, support weight management, promote better focus and productivity, and contribute to improved overall well-being. Whether you're a busy professional, a parent on-the-go, or an athlete seeking post-workout nourishment, balanced snacks can be your ally in achieving your health and lifestyle goals.

Discover the magic of pairing fruits with proteins, vegetables with healthy fats, and whole grains with nutrient-dense toppings. We've curated an array of mouthwatering snack ideas that will not only satisfy your taste buds but also provide your body with the essential nutrients it needs to thrive.

Balanced snacks that combine carbohydrates, proteins, and fats offer several benefits:

- **Sustained Energy:** Carbohydrates provide a quick source of energy, while proteins and fats slow down digestion, providing lasting energy.
- **Blood Sugar Control:** Balanced snacks help stabilize blood sugar levels, preventing energy crashes and sudden hunger.
- **Improved Satiety:** The combination of nutrients in balanced snacks keeps you feeling full and satisfied, reducing the likelihood of overeating later.

Nourishing Snack Ideas: Wholesome and Delicious Choices for Every Palate

Snacking is an integral part of our daily lives, providing a much-needed energy boost and satisfying our cravings between meals.

However, it can be challenging to find snacks that are both nourishing and delicious. That's where this guide comes in.

We have curated a diverse selection of nourishing snack ideas that cater to different taste preferences, dietary needs, and lifestyles.

In today's fast-paced world, it's essential to choose snacks that not only provide quick energy but also offer a wealth of essential nutrients to support overall health and well-being.

Whether you're looking for a post-workout refuel, an afternoon pick-me-up, or a guilt-free indulgence, our snack ideas have got you covered.

From sweet to savory, crunchy to creamy, and everything in between, we have carefully selected a variety of snack options to delight your taste buds and keep you feeling satisfied.

These snacks are designed to be balanced, incorporating the right combination of macronutrients to stabilize blood sugar levels and provide sustained energy throughout the day.

In this guide, you will discover easy-to-prepare snack ideas that are packed with nutrient-dense ingredients like fruits, vegetables, nuts, seeds, and lean proteins.

We've also included options for those with dietary restrictions, such as gluten-free, vegan, and low-carb snacks, so everyone can find a snack that suits their needs.

Embrace the joy of snacking with our nourishing snack ideas and savor every bite knowing that you are fueling your body with wholesome goodness.

Let's embark on a flavorful journey of delicious and satisfying snacks that will nourish your body and delight your taste buds, ensuring that your snacking experience is not only enjoyable but also beneficial for your overall well-being.

1. Apple Slices with Almond Butter: Enjoy the natural sweetness of apple slices paired with the richness of almond butter, which provides protein and healthy fats.

2. Greek Yogurt Parfait: Layer Greek yogurt with fresh berries, nuts, and a drizzle of honey for a protein-packed and antioxidant-rich snack.

3. Veggie Sticks with Hummus: Dip crunchy vegetable sticks like carrots, cucumber, and bell peppers into hummus for a satisfying and fiber-filled snack.

4. Trail Mix: Create a custom trail mix with a mix of nuts, seeds, dried fruits, and dark chocolate for a balanced blend of flavors and textures.

5. Avocado Toast: Top whole-grain toast with mashed avocado, cherry tomatoes, and a sprinkle of salt and pepper for a creamy and nutritious snack.

6. Rice Cakes with Cottage Cheese and Berries: Spread cottage cheese over rice cakes and top with fresh berries for a protein-rich and refreshing snack.

7. Energy Bites: Make homemade energy bites using oats, nut butter, honey, and seeds. These portable treats are great for on-the-go snacking.

8. Popcorn with Nutritional Yeast: Sprinkle nutritional yeast over air-popped popcorn for a savory and satisfying snack.

9. Smoothie Bowl: Blend a smoothie with your favorite fruits and veggies, then top it with granola, nuts, and seeds for added crunch and nutrition.

10. Whole Fruit with Cheese: Pair whole fruits like apple slices or grapes with a small serving of cheese for a delightful combination of flavors.

11. Cottage Cheese with Pineapple: Enjoy the sweetness of pineapple combined with protein-packed cottage cheese for a tropical-inspired snack.

12. Cucumber and Tuna Bites: Top cucumber slices with canned tuna and a dollop of Greek yogurt for a refreshing and protein-rich snack.

13. Roasted Chickpeas: Toss chickpeas in olive oil and your favorite spices, then roast them until crispy for a satisfying and crunchy snack.

14. Rice Paper Rolls: Fill rice paper with shredded veggies, cooked shrimp or tofu, and herbs for a light and refreshing snack.

15. Nut Butter and Banana Sandwich: Spread nut butter between banana slices for a quick and nutrient-rich snack.

16. Edamame: Enjoy a bowl of steamed edamame with a sprinkle of sea salt for a protein-rich and satisfying snack.

17. Stuffed Bell Pepper: Fill bell pepper halves with a mixture of quinoa, beans, and spices, then bake until tender and delicious.

18. Veggie Chips: Bake thinly sliced vegetables like sweet potatoes, beets, or zucchini for a healthier alternative to potato chips.

19. Greek Yogurt with Chia Seeds: Top Greek yogurt with chia seeds and your favorite fruits for a creamy and nutritious snack.

20. Chia Seed Pudding: Mix chia seeds with almond milk and your favorite flavors like cocoa or vanilla for a delicious and nutritious pudding.

Incorporating a variety of nourishing snacks into your daily routine can promote sustained energy, keep you satisfied between meals, and contribute to a balanced and wholesome diet. Whether you prefer sweet or savory, crunchy or creamy, these snack ideas offer something for everyone's taste preferences and dietary needs. Remember to listen to your body's hunger cues and enjoy snacks mindfully to fully appreciate their flavors and benefits. By making nourishing snacking a part of your lifestyle, you can support your overall health and well-being while indulging in delicious and satisfying treats throughout the day.

Chapter Eight

Vegan and Vegetarian Delights: A Wholesome Journey into Plant-Based Culinary Bliss

In recent years, the popularity of vegan and vegetarian diets has soared as more individuals embrace a compassionate, sustainable, and health-conscious approach to eating. These plant-based lifestyles offer a wide array of delicious and nutritious options that cater to different taste preferences, dietary needs, and ethical beliefs. From colorful salads to hearty grain bowls, plant-based cuisines are celebrated for their abundance of flavors, textures, and health benefits.

This comprehensive guide explores the diverse world of vegan and vegetarian delights, delving into the principles of plant-based eating, the health benefits associated with these diets, and a plethora of mouthwatering recipes that will satisfy even the most discerning palates.

Whether you're a seasoned vegan, a curious vegetarian, or simply looking to incorporate more plant-based meals into your diet, this guide has something for everyone.

Understanding Vegan and Vegetarian Diets: Embracing Plant-Based Lifestyles for Health and Compassion

Vegan and vegetarian diets are plant-based eating patterns that have gained significant popularity in recent years due to their numerous health benefits, ethical considerations, and environmental consciousness. Both diets center around a predominantly plant-based approach, emphasizing a wide variety of fruits, vegetables, grains, legumes, nuts, and seeds.

However, there are fundamental differences between the two in terms of the inclusion of animal-derived products.

Vegan Diet:

A vegan diet is a fully plant-based diet that excludes all animal-derived foods, including meat (red meat, poultry, and seafood), dairy products (milk, cheese, yogurt, butter), eggs, and honey.

Vegans abstain from using animal-based ingredients in all aspects of life, extending beyond just dietary choices. The primary focus of a vegan lifestyle is rooted in compassion for animals, promoting animal welfare, and reducing the environmental impact of animal agriculture.

Vegetarian Diet:

A vegetarian diet, on the other hand, excludes meat (red meat, poultry, and seafood) but may include animal-derived products like dairy and eggs.

The classification of vegetarians varies based on the inclusion or exclusion of specific animal products:

a. Lacto-vegetarians eat dairy foods but stay away from meat and eggs.

b. Ovo-vegetarian diets include eggs but do not include meat or dairy products.

c. vegetarian diet that includes dairy products and eggs but excludes meat.

Health Benefits of Vegan and Vegetarian Diets

Both vegan and vegetarian diets offer numerous health benefits, including:

1. Lower Risk of Chronic Diseases: Plant-based diets have been associated with a reduced risk of heart disease, certain cancers, type 2 diabetes, and hypertension.

2. Weight Management: Plant-based diets are often lower in calories and saturated fat, making them conducive to weight management and weight loss.

3. Improved Digestive Health: The high fiber content in plant-based foods supports a healthy digestive system and may reduce the risk of digestive issues.

4. Nutrient-Rich: Plant-based diets are rich in essential nutrients such as vitamins, minerals, fiber, and antioxidants that promote overall well-being.

5. Better Blood Sugar Control: Plant-based diets can help manage blood sugar levels, making them beneficial for individuals with diabetes.

Vegan and vegetarian diets are driven by ethical considerations:

1. Animal Welfare: Vegans choose a cruelty-free lifestyle to promote the ethical treatment of animals and to avoid supporting industries involved in animal exploitation.

2. Environmental Impact: Both diets aim to reduce the environmental footprint associated with animal agriculture, which is a significant contributor to greenhouse gas emissions and deforestation.

3. Sustainable Living: Plant-based diets support sustainable living by utilizing fewer resources like water and land, making them environmentally friendly choices.

Adopting a Vegan or Vegetarian Lifestyle
Switching to a vegan or vegetarian lifestyle requires careful consideration and planning to ensure proper nutrient intake. Individuals should be mindful of essential nutrients such as protein, iron, vitamin B12, omega-3 fatty acids, calcium, and vitamin D,

which may need to be obtained from plant-based sources or supplements.

Ultimately, embracing a vegan or vegetarian lifestyle represents a commitment to making conscious and compassionate choices that benefit personal health, animal welfare, and the planet. By understanding the principles and benefits of these diets, individuals can make informed decisions to embark on a journey of plant-based eating that aligns with their values and health goals.

Embracing a Plant-Based Lifestyle

1. Plant Protein Sources: Discover a diverse range of plant-based protein sources such as legumes (beans, lentils, chickpeas), tofu, tempeh, edamame, quinoa, and nuts.

2. Plant Milk Alternatives: Explore various plant-based milk alternatives like almond milk, soy milk, oat milk, coconut milk, and rice milk.

3. Cooking Techniques: Learn about different cooking techniques to elevate the flavors of plant-based dishes, from roasting and grilling to sautéing and steaming.

4. Essential Nutrients: Understand the importance of key nutrients in plant-based diets, including iron, calcium, vitamin B12, omega-3 fatty acids, and vitamin D.

5. Meal Planning: Master the art of meal planning for vegan and vegetarian diets, ensuring balanced and satisfying meals throughout the week.

Delightful Vegan and Vegetarian Recipes

1. Hearty Grain Bowls: Wholesome bowls filled with quinoa, brown rice, roasted vegetables, and protein-rich legumes.

2. Flavorful Curries: Aromatic and vibrant curries featuring a medley of vegetables and tofu or chickpeas in creamy coconut milk.

3. Plant-Based Burgers: Mouthwatering veggie burgers made with black beans, lentils, mushrooms, or beets, accompanied by creative toppings and sauces.

4. Fresh Salads: Refreshing salads with a mix of leafy greens, colorful vegetables, nuts, seeds, and homemade dressings.

5. Nourishing Soups: Comforting soups packed with nutrient-dense ingredients like lentils, sweet potatoes, and leafy greens.

6. Stir-Fries: Quick and colorful stir-fries featuring an array of vegetables, tofu, or tempeh in flavorful sauces.

7. Decadent Desserts: Indulgent vegan desserts like rich chocolate avocado mousse, dairy-free ice cream, and delectable fruit-based treats.

Navigating Vegan and Vegetarian Cuisine

1. Eating Out: Discover tips for dining out at restaurants and navigating plant-based options on menus.

2. Vegan-Friendly Travel: Learn how to maintain a plant-based lifestyle while traveling and exploring new destinations.

3. Family-Friendly Meals: Plan vegan and vegetarian meals that cater to the tastes of the whole family.

4. Special Occasions: Create delicious plant-based dishes for holidays, parties, and special celebrations.

The Ethics of Plant-Based Eating

1. Environmental Impact: Explore the positive impact of plant-based diets on the environment, including reduced greenhouse gas emissions and water usage.

2. Animal Welfare: Understand how a vegan lifestyle aligns with principles of compassion and kindness towards animals.

3. Sustainable Practices: Embrace sustainable practices like local and seasonal eating to support the planet and local communities.

Embracing a vegan or vegetarian lifestyle opens up a world of delectable possibilities, allowing individuals to savor the flavors of plant-based cuisines while supporting their health, the environment, and animal welfare.

With this comprehensive guide, you'll embark on a fulfilling and nourishing journey into the realm of vegan and vegetarian delights, unlocking a vibrant tapestry of plant-based culinary bliss for your enjoyment and well-being.

Whether you're looking for a new way of eating or seeking to expand your plant-based repertoire, this guide is your gateway to a world of wholesome, delicious, and compassionate meals.

Chapter Nine

Protein-Rich Dishes: Nourishing Kidney Health with Flavor and Balance

Protein-rich dishes are an essential aspect of a balanced diet, providing our bodies with the building blocks for tissue repair, immune function, and various other physiological processes.
However, for individuals with kidney health concerns, such as chronic kidney disease (CKD), managing protein intake becomes even more critical. This comprehensive guide delves into the importance of protein in kidney health, the challenges faced by those with kidney disease, and a diverse range of delicious and kidney-friendly protein-rich dishes that promote overall well-being.

The Role of Protein in Kidney Health: A Vital Nutrient for Balance and Function

Protein plays a crucial role in maintaining kidney health and supporting various essential functions within the body. As one of the three macronutrients (alongside carbohydrates and fats), protein serves as the building block for tissues, enzymes, hormones, and other essential molecules.

However, in the context of kidney health, the role of protein becomes particularly important as the kidneys play a significant role in processing and excreting waste products generated from protein metabolism.

Key Aspects of the Role of Protein in Kidney Health:

1. Tissue Repair and Growth: Proteins are composed of amino acids, which are essential for repairing damaged tissues and supporting the growth of new cells.

2. Enzymes and Hormones: Many enzymes and hormones responsible for essential bodily processes are composed of protein.

3. Immune Function: Proteins are vital for maintaining a healthy immune system, helping the body defend against infections and diseases.

4. Fluid Balance: Proteins are involved in maintaining fluid balance within the body, ensuring that fluids are distributed appropriately between cells and blood vessels.

5. Acid-Base Balance: Proteins help regulate the body's pH levels, maintaining a stable acid-base balance.

6. Transport and Storage: Proteins aid in the transport of nutrients, oxygen, and waste products throughout the body, as well as the storage of important molecules.

7. Muscle Health: Proteins are crucial for maintaining muscle health and strength.

Protein and Kidney Health:
For individuals with healthy kidneys, consuming an adequate amount of protein is generally beneficial for overall health and well-being.

However, for those with kidney health concerns, such as chronic kidney disease (CKD), the role of protein requires careful consideration.

1. Kidney Filtration: The kidneys play a vital role in filtering waste products from the blood. Protein metabolism produces waste products like urea and creatinine, which are normally excreted in the urine by healthy kidneys.

2. Protein Waste Accumulation: In individuals with impaired kidney function, the kidneys may struggle to filter and excrete these waste products, leading to their accumulation in the bloodstream.

3. Proteinuria: Excessive protein intake may lead to proteinuria, a condition where excess protein is excreted in the urine, indicating potential kidney damage.

4. Protein-Energy Wasting: In advanced stages of CKD, a condition known as protein-energy wasting may occur, leading to muscle loss, malnutrition, and overall poor health.

Balancing Protein Intake for Kidney Health:
For individuals with kidney health concerns, it is essential to strike a balance between obtaining enough protein for necessary bodily functions while

avoiding excessive protein intake that may strain the kidneys.

1. High-Quality Proteins: Focus on consuming high-quality proteins that contain all essential amino acids and are easily digestible, such as lean meats, poultry, fish, eggs, and plant-based sources like tofu and quinoa.

2. Individualized Approach: Work closely with healthcare providers and registered dietitians to determine the appropriate amount of protein intake based on individual health needs, kidney function, and overall well-being.

3. Protein Distribution: Distribute protein intake evenly throughout the day to avoid consuming large amounts in one sitting.

4. Monitoring Proteinuria: Regularly monitor protein excretion in the urine to assess the effectiveness of protein management.

By understanding the role of protein in kidney health and adopting a mindful approach to protein intake, individuals can support their kidney function while still obtaining the essential nutrients necessary for overall health and vitality.

It is crucial for individuals with kidney health concerns to work closely with healthcare professionals to tailor their protein intake to their specific needs and medical conditions.

Kidney-Friendly Protein-Rich Dishes

1. Grilled Lemon Herb Chicken: Flavorful chicken marinated with herbs and lemon juice, grilled to perfection.

2. Baked Salmon with Herbs: Nutrient-rich salmon seasoned with fresh herbs and baked to tender perfection.

3. Tofu Stir-Fry with Vegetables: Stir-fried tofu and a variety of colorful vegetables seasoned with savory sauces.

4. Quinoa and Black Bean Salad: A satisfying salad with protein-packed quinoa, black beans, and a medley of vegetables.

5. Lentil and Vegetable Soup: Hearty soup with protein-rich lentils, vegetables, and aromatic spices.

6. Egg White Omelette: Fluffy egg white omelette filled with nutritious vegetables and low-fat cheese.

7. Greek Yogurt Parfait: Creamy Greek yogurt layered with fresh fruits and a sprinkling of nuts or seeds.

8. Chickpea and Vegetable Curry: A flavorful curry featuring chickpeas and a blend of aromatic spices and vegetables.

9. Baked Falafel: Baked falafel patties made from ground chickpeas and herbs, served with a refreshing tahini sauce.

10. Quinoa Stuffed Bell Peppers: Bell peppers filled with protein-rich quinoa, vegetables, and herbs, baked to perfection.

11. Lentil and Mushroom Bolognese: A hearty pasta dish featuring lentils and mushrooms in a rich tomato sauce.

12. Black Bean Tacos: Tasty tacos filled with seasoned black beans, fresh salsa, and avocado slices.

13. Mediterranean Tofu Skewers: Marinated tofu cubes threaded onto skewers and grilled to a delightful texture.

14. Eggplant and Chickpea Tagine: A Moroccan-inspired tagine featuring tender eggplant and chickpeas in a spiced tomato sauce.

15. Cauliflower Rice and Pea Pilaf: A light and flavorful pilaf made with cauliflower rice, green peas, and fragrant spices.

Snacks and Desserts for Kidney Health:
1. Roasted Chickpeas: Crunchy and protein-packed chickpeas roasted with savory spices.
2. Greek Yogurt with Berries: Creamy Greek yogurt topped with fresh berries for a satisfying snack.
3. Almond Butter Energy Bites: Nutrient-dense bites made with almond butter, oats, and seeds.
4. Chia Seed Pudding: A nutritious and delicious pudding made with chia seeds and almond milk.
5. Baked Apple Chips: Thin slices of apples baked to a crisp, sweet treat.
6. Trail Mix: A mix of nuts, seeds, and dried fruits for a wholesome and portable snack.
7. Dark Chocolate-Dipped Strawberries: Sweet strawberries dipped in dark chocolate for an indulgent dessert.

Embracing a Kidney-Friendly Protein-Rich Diet:
1. Meal Planning: Plan balanced and kidney-friendly meals that incorporate the right amount of protein and essential nutrients.

2. Hydration: Stay hydrated to support kidney function and help prevent dehydration.

3. Regular Monitoring: Regularly monitor kidney function and proteinuria with the guidance of healthcare providers.

4. Lifestyle Factors: Adopt a healthy lifestyle with regular physical activity and avoiding smoking and excessive alcohol consumption.

5. Individualized Approach: Work closely with healthcare providers and registered dietitians to tailor dietary plans based on individual health needs and kidney function.

By understanding the importance of protein in kidney health and adopting a mindful approach to protein management, individuals can continue to enjoy delicious and nutritious protein-rich dishes while supporting their kidney health.

With a variety of flavorful recipes and careful consideration of dietary needs, nourishing the body and promoting kidney well-being can be a delightful journey into the world of protein-rich culinary delights.

Chapter Ten

Heart-Healthy Fats and Diabetes Management: Nurturing Cardiovascular Health and Glucose Control

Diabetes management is a delicate balance that involves monitoring blood sugar levels, making mindful dietary choices, and maintaining a heart-healthy lifestyle. Among the various dietary components, fats play a crucial role in diabetes management and cardiovascular health. Understanding the types of fats and their impact on blood sugar levels and heart health is vital for individuals with diabetes. This comprehensive guide explores the role of heart-healthy fats in diabetes management, the relationship between diabetes and cardiovascular health, and a diverse range of delicious and nutritious recipes that promote both glucose control and heart well-being.

While managing carbohydrate intake is vital for blood sugar control, the type and quantity of dietary fats are equally important.

Heart-healthy fats, also known as unsaturated fats, have been shown to offer several health benefits, including:

1. Cardiovascular Health: Unsaturated fats can help improve cholesterol levels, reduce inflammation, and lower the risk of heart disease, which is a common complication of diabetes.

2. Blood Sugar Control: Consuming heart-healthy fats in combination with carbohydrates can slow down the absorption of glucose, leading to better blood sugar management.

3. Satiety and Weight Management: Fats are more calorie-dense than carbohydrates or protein, providing a sense of fullness and satisfaction, which may aid in weight management.

Types of Heart-Healthy Fats

1. Monounsaturated Fats: Found in foods such as olive oil, avocados, nuts, and seeds, monounsaturated fats have been associated with improved heart health and blood sugar control.

2. Polyunsaturated Fats: These fats are found in fatty fish (salmon, mackerel, sardines), flaxseeds, chia seeds, and walnuts. Polyunsaturated fats contain essential omega-3 and omega-6 fatty acids, which are important for heart and brain health.

3. Omega-3 Fatty Acids: A subgroup of polyunsaturated fats, omega-3s have been shown to reduce inflammation, lower triglycerides, and support heart health. They are abundant in fatty fish, flaxseeds, chia seeds, and walnuts.

4. Omega-6 Fatty Acids: Another subgroup of polyunsaturated fats, omega-6s play a role in promoting heart health and are found in vegetable oils, nuts, and seeds.

5. Plant Sterols and Stanols: These naturally occurring substances found in plant-based foods can help lower LDL (bad) cholesterol levels.

Managing Dietary Fats for Diabetes Management:

1. Replacing Saturated Fats: Minimize consumption of saturated fats found in red meat, full-fat dairy, and processed foods, as they can raise LDL cholesterol levels and increase the risk of heart disease.

2. Limiting Trans Fats: Avoid trans fats, which are artificial fats found in partially hydrogenated oils, as they have been linked to adverse heart health and inflammation.

3. Moderation and Portion Control: While heart-healthy fats have numerous benefits, they are calorie-dense. Practice portion control to manage caloric intake.

4. Cooking Methods: Opt for heart-healthy cooking methods like baking, grilling, steaming, and sautéing with minimal oil to reduce saturated fat consumption.

The Connection Between Diabetes and Cardiovascular Health:

Individuals with diabetes are at a higher risk of developing cardiovascular disease, which includes heart attacks, strokes, and other heart-related complications.

The connection between diabetes and cardiovascular health can be attributed to various factors, including:

1. Insulin Resistance: Insulin resistance, a hallmark of type 2 diabetes, can promote inflammation and damage blood vessels, leading to cardiovascular issues.

2. High Blood Sugar Levels: Prolonged elevated blood sugar levels can damage blood vessels and contribute to atherosclerosis, a condition characterized by plaque buildup in the arteries.

3. High Blood Pressure: Hypertension, often associated with diabetes, puts additional strain on the heart and blood vessels, increasing the risk of heart disease.

4. High Cholesterol Levels: Uncontrolled diabetes can lead to abnormal cholesterol levels, increasing the likelihood of heart problems.

5. Obesity: Obesity, a common risk factor for type 2 diabetes, is also associated with an increased risk of cardiovascular disease.

By managing blood sugar levels and adopting a heart-healthy lifestyle that includes a balanced intake of heart-healthy fats, individuals with diabetes can reduce their risk of developing cardiovascular complications and enhance overall well-being.

1. Avocado and Tomato Salad: A refreshing salad featuring avocado, cherry tomatoes, cucumbers, and a zesty lemon vinaigrette.

2. Baked Salmon with Lemon-Dill Sauce: Heart-healthy omega-3-rich salmon baked to perfection, served with a light lemon-dill sauce.

3. Grilled Mediterranean Vegetable Skewers: Colorful skewers loaded with bell peppers, zucchini, cherry tomatoes, and red onions, seasoned with herbs and olive oil.

4. Quinoa and Chickpea Salad: A protein-packed salad featuring quinoa, chickpeas, fresh herbs, and a lemon-tahini dressing.

5. Walnut-Crusted Chicken Tenders: Tender chicken tenders coated with crushed walnuts and baked to a crunchy perfection.

6. Flaxseed and Berry Smoothie: A nutrient-dense smoothie made with flaxseeds, mixed berries, Greek yogurt, and a touch of honey.

7. Spinach and Mushroom Stuffed Bell Peppers: Bell peppers filled with a savory mixture of spinach, mushrooms, brown rice, and mozzarella cheese.

8. Pistachio-Crusted Cod: A delightful fish dish featuring pistachio-crusted cod fillets served with a lemon-butter sauce.

9. Chia Seed Pudding Parfait: A delicious and satisfying parfait made with chia seed pudding, Greek yogurt, and layers of fresh berries.

10. Broccoli and Almond Salad: A vibrant salad combining steamed broccoli, toasted almonds, dried cranberries, and a tangy balsamic vinaigrette.

11. Sautéed Garlic Shrimp with Asparagus: Succulent shrimp and crisp asparagus sautéed in garlic-infused olive oil.

12. Tofu and Vegetable Stir-Fry: A plant-based stir-fry featuring tofu, colorful vegetables, and a savory soy-ginger sauce.

13. Pecan-Crusted Sweet Potato Wedges: Sweet potato wedges coated with crushed pecans and baked to a delightful crisp.

14. Baked Mediterranean Chicken: Tender chicken thighs marinated in Mediterranean-inspired spices, baked with olives, tomatoes, and feta cheese.

15. Berry and Walnut Spinach Salad: A nutrient-rich salad with fresh spinach, mixed berries, goat cheese, and toasted walnuts, drizzled with balsamic vinaigrette.

By incorporating heart-healthy fats and a wide array of nutrient-dense recipes into their diets, individuals with diabetes can manage their blood sugar levels effectively and promote cardiovascular health.
With the right knowledge and culinary inspiration, individuals can embark on a journey of culinary delights that nourish both body and heart, enhancing their diabetes management and overall well-being.

Chapter Eleven

Low Sodium and Kidney-Friendly Recipes: Flavorful Delights for Optimal Kidney Health

A low sodium diet is essential for individuals with kidney health concerns, especially those with chronic kidney disease (CKD). Managing sodium intake helps maintain fluid balance and blood pressure, reducing the strain on the kidneys.

This comprehensive guide explores the importance of a low sodium and kidney-friendly diet, the relationship between sodium and kidney health, and a diverse range of delicious and nutritious recipes that cater to optimal kidney health.

The Role of Sodium in Kidney Health:
Sodium, a mineral commonly found in salt and processed foods, is essential for various bodily functions, including maintaining fluid balance,

transmitting nerve signals, and supporting muscle function.

However, excessive sodium intake can be detrimental to kidney health, especially for those with compromised kidney function.

The kidneys play a crucial role in filtering excess sodium and maintaining a delicate balance of sodium and water in the body.

Challenges in Sodium Management for Kidney Health:

1. Fluid Retention: Consuming too much sodium can lead to fluid retention, putting extra strain on the kidneys and increasing the risk of edema (swelling).

2. High Blood Pressure: Excessive sodium intake can raise blood pressure, which is a risk factor for kidney disease and cardiovascular issues.

3. Progression of CKD: In individuals with CKD, a high sodium diet may accelerate the progression of kidney damage.

4. Electrolyte Imbalance: Imbalanced sodium levels can disrupt other electrolytes in the body, leading to complications like hyperkalemia (high potassium) and hyponatremia (low sodium).

Importance of a Low Sodium Diet for Kidney Health:

1. Blood Pressure Management: Reducing sodium intake helps regulate blood pressure, benefiting both kidney health and overall cardiovascular well-being.

2. Fluid Balance: Limiting sodium helps control fluid retention, preventing edema and maintaining proper hydration.

3. Slowing CKD Progression: A low sodium diet may help slow the progression of CKD and preserve kidney function.

4. Supporting Medication Efficacy: Lowering sodium intake can enhance the effectiveness of blood pressure medications and other treatments.

Recommended Sodium Intake:

For individuals with kidney health concerns, it is essential to follow a low sodium diet. The recommended daily intake of sodium for the general population is around 2,300 milligrams (mg), but for individuals with kidney disease, healthcare providers may recommend even lower sodium levels, typically ranging from 1,500 to 2,000 mg per day.

Tips for Reducing Sodium Intake

1. Choose Fresh and Unprocessed Foods: Opt for fresh fruits, vegetables, and whole grains rather than processed and packaged foods, which are typically high in sodium.

2. Read Food Labels: Pay attention to sodium content on food labels and choose products with lower sodium levels.

3. Limit the Use of Salt: Reduce the amount of salt used in cooking and at the table. Experiment with herbs, spices, and citrus flavors to enhance taste without added sodium.

4. Be Wary of Condiments: Many condiments include a lot of sodium, including ketchup, soy sauce, and salad dressings. Use them sparingly or look for alternatives that are low in salt.

5. Rinse Canned Foods: If using canned vegetables or beans, rinse them thoroughly to reduce their sodium content.

6. Avoid High-Sodium Seasonings: Some seasoning blends and bouillon cubes can be high in sodium. Opt for low sodium or sodium-free versions.

Kidney-Friendly Recipes for Optimal Kidney Health

1. Lemon Herb Baked Chicken: Tender chicken breasts marinated in lemon juice, garlic, and herbs, baked to perfection.

2. Grilled Vegetable Skewers: Colorful vegetable skewers featuring bell peppers, zucchini, and mushrooms, lightly seasoned and grilled to enhance flavor.

3. Quinoa and Black Bean Salad: A protein-packed salad with quinoa, black beans, cherry tomatoes, and a tangy lime vinaigrette.

4. Baked Salmon with Dill Sauce: Heart-healthy salmon fillets baked with a creamy dill sauce made with Greek yogurt.

5. Zucchini Noodles with Tomato Sauce: Zucchini noodles (zoodles) served with a flavorful and low sodium tomato sauce.

6. Spinach and Feta Stuffed Bell Peppers: Bell peppers filled with a delicious mixture of spinach, feta cheese, and quinoa.

7. Mediterranean Chickpea Salad: A refreshing salad featuring chickpeas, cucumbers, cherry tomatoes, olives, and a lemon-herb dressing.

8. Cilantro Lime Shrimp Tacos: Succulent shrimp marinated in cilantro and lime, served in soft corn tortillas with fresh salsa.

9. Lentil and Vegetable Soup: A comforting and nourishing soup made with lentils, carrots, celery, and a blend of herbs and spices.

10. Eggplant and Chickpea Curry: A flavorful curry featuring eggplant, chickpeas, and a fragrant blend of spices.

11. Herbed Quinoa Pilaf: Quinoa cooked with a mix of fresh herbs and vegetables, creating a flavorful and nutritious side dish.

12. Greek Yogurt Parfait with Berries: Creamy Greek yogurt layered with fresh berries and a sprinkle of granola for added crunch.

13. Stuffed Portobello Mushrooms: Portobello mushrooms stuffed with a savory mixture of quinoa, spinach, and feta cheese.

14. Turkey and Vegetable Stir-Fry: Lean turkey breast and a medley of colorful vegetables stir-fried with a low sodium sauce.

15. Baked Sweet Potato Fries: Sweet potato fries baked to a crispy texture and seasoned with herbs and spices.

Incorporating these low sodium and kidney-friendly recipes into the diet can promote optimal kidney health while providing delicious and satisfying meals.

It is essential for individuals with kidney health concerns to work closely with healthcare providers and registered dietitians to develop a personalized low sodium meal plan that caters to their specific health needs and supports kidney function.

By adopting a mindful approach to sodium intake and embracing a variety of flavorful recipes, individuals can enhance their kidney health and overall well-being.

Chapter Twelve

Creative Substitutions for Special Diets: Navigating Dietary Restrictions with Flavor and Variety

Special diets are often necessary to address specific health concerns, food allergies, intolerances, or ethical considerations. Whether you are following a gluten-free, dairy-free, vegetarian, vegan, or other special diet, finding creative substitutions is essential to maintain a balanced and enjoyable eating experience.

This comprehensive guide explores the importance of special diets, common dietary restrictions, and a diverse range of creative substitutions that cater to different dietary needs while providing flavor and variety.

Understanding the Importance of Special Diets:
Special diets are not only about restrictions; they are about nourishing the body and promoting overall well-being.

For individuals with health conditions like celiac disease, lactose intolerance, diabetes, or food allergies, adhering to a special diet can significantly improve their quality of life and manage their health effectively.

Additionally, special diets can be a personal choice driven by ethical, environmental, or cultural considerations.

Common Special Diets and Dietary Restrictions

1. Gluten-Free Diet: A gluten-free diet excludes gluten, a protein found in wheat, barley, rye, and their derivatives. For those who have celiac disease or gluten intolerance, it is crucial.

2. Dairy-Free Diet: A dairy-free diet excludes all dairy products, often due to lactose intolerance or milk allergies.

3. Vegetarian Diet: A vegetarian diet excludes meat, poultry, and fish, but may include dairy and eggs.

4. Vegan Diet: A vegan diet excludes all animal products, including meat, dairy, eggs, and any other animal-derived ingredients.

5. Paleo Diet: The paleo diet focuses on whole foods and excludes processed foods, grains, legumes, and dairy, mimicking the presumed diet of our ancestors.

6. Ketogenic Diet: A low-carb, high-fat diet that induces ketosis and is often used for weight loss or managing epilepsy.

7. Low-FODMAP Diet: This diet restricts certain fermentable carbohydrates to manage irritable bowel syndrome (IBS) symptoms.

8. Low Sodium Diet: A low sodium diet restricts salt intake to manage blood pressure and kidney health.

9. Diabetes Diet: A balanced diet that focuses on controlling carbohydrate intake to manage blood sugar levels in individuals with diabetes.

1. Gluten-Free Flour Alternatives: Substitute wheat flour with gluten-free flours like almond flour, coconut flour, rice flour, or a gluten-free baking blend for baking and cooking.

2. Dairy-Free Milk Alternatives: Replace cow's milk with plant-based milk alternatives like almond, soy, oat, or coconut milk.

3. Plant-Based Proteins: For vegetarian and vegan diets, opt for plant-based protein sources like beans, lentils, tofu, tempeh, quinoa, and edamame.

4. Vegan Butter and Spreads: Use vegan butter, avocado, or nut butter as dairy-free alternatives for spreading and cooking.

5. Egg Replacements: For vegan baking, use flaxseed meal, chia seeds, applesauce, or mashed bananas as egg replacements.

6. Vegetable Noodles: Replace traditional pasta with zucchini noodles (zoodles), sweet potato noodles, or spaghetti squash for a lower-carb option.

7. Nutritional Yeast: A vegan alternative to cheese, nutritional yeast provides a cheesy flavor and is a good source of B vitamins.

8. Cauliflower Rice: Swap rice with cauliflower rice for a low-carb and nutrient-rich alternative.

9. Coconut Aminos: Use coconut aminos as a gluten-free and lower-sodium alternative to soy sauce.

10. Date Paste: A natural sweetener made from dates, date paste can replace refined sugars in recipes.

11. Avocado as Butter Replacement: Use mashed avocado as a butter substitute in baking for added moisture and healthy fats.

12. Vegetable Broths: Opt for vegetable broth as a flavorful and lower-sodium alternative to meat-based broths.

13. Coconut Cream: Replace heavy cream with coconut cream for dairy-free creaminess in recipes.

14. Chia Seeds as Thickener: Chia seeds can be used as a thickening agent in recipes instead of eggs or gelatin.

15. Spaghetti Squash as Pasta: Cooked spaghetti squash makes an excellent substitute for traditional pasta.

1. Gluten-Free Banana Bread: A delicious gluten-free and dairy-free version of classic banana bread made with almond flour and coconut oil.

2. Vegan Cauliflower Buffalo Wings: Cauliflower florets coated in a crispy gluten-free batter and tossed in buffalo sauce for a vegan take on classic buffalo wings.

3. Dairy-Free Mac and Cheese: Creamy macaroni and cheese made with a dairy-free cheese sauce using nutritional yeast and plant-based milk.

4. Vegetarian Lentil Shepherd's Pie: A hearty and comforting dish made with lentils, vegetables, and a mashed potato topping.

5. Vegan Chocolate Avocado Mousse: A rich and indulgent chocolate mousse made with ripe avocados and plant-based milk.

6. Low-Carb Eggplant Lasagna: Layers of thinly sliced eggplant, marinara sauce, and plant-based cheese for a low-carb lasagna option.

7. Grain-Free Pizza Crust: A grain-free pizza crust made with cauliflower or almond flour, topped with dairy-free cheese and vegetable toppings.

8. Vegan Quinoa Stuffed Bell Peppers: Bell peppers filled with a flavorful mixture of quinoa, black beans, and spices.

9. Dairy-Free Spinach and Artichoke Dip: A creamy and dairy-free version of the classic spinach and artichoke dip using cashews and nutritional yeast.

10. Keto Avocado Bacon Burger: A juicy burger topped with avocado, bacon, and lettuce wrapped in lettuce leaves instead of a bun for a keto-friendly option.

11. Low-FODMAP Stir-Fry: A colorful stir-fry with low-FODMAP vegetables, tofu or chicken, and a simple soy sauce replacement.

12. Diabetic-Friendly Cauliflower Fried Rice: A low-carb version of fried rice using cauliflower rice, vegetables, and lean protein.

13. Vegan Coconut Curry: A flavorful and creamy coconut curry made with tofu or vegetables and served with cauliflower rice.

14. Low Sodium Lemon Herb Chicken: Tender chicken breasts marinated in a lemon-herb sauce with no added salt.

15. Dairy-Free Mango Smoothie: A refreshing smoothie made with coconut milk, fresh mango, and a touch of honey or maple syrup.

Creative substitutions and recipes provide an array of options for individuals with special dietary needs, offering delicious and nutritious alternatives to traditional dishes.

Embracing creativity and exploring new ingredients can lead to exciting culinary adventures while supporting optimal health and dietary goals.

When adopting a special diet, it is essential to consult with healthcare providers or registered dietitians to ensure nutritional needs are met and dietary requirements are appropriately addressed.

By incorporating creative substitutions and diverse recipes, individuals can enjoy a varied and satisfying eating experience that caters to their unique dietary needs and enhances their overall well-being.

Chapter Thirteen

Desserts: Sweet Treats with Diabetes in Mind

Managing diabetes doesn't mean giving up on sweet treats. With a mindful approach and creative ingredient choices, individuals with diabetes can enjoy delicious desserts without compromising their blood sugar control. This comprehensive guide explores the role of desserts in diabetes management, the impact of different sweeteners on blood sugar levels, and a diverse range of diabetes-friendly dessert recipes that cater to those with a sweet tooth while considering their nutritional needs.

Understanding the Role of Desserts in Diabetes Management

Desserts often evoke feelings of indulgence and celebration, but for individuals with diabetes, it can be challenging to navigate their sweet cravings while maintaining stable blood sugar levels.

Desserts can be a part of a balanced diet for individuals with diabetes, but it's essential to choose wisely and manage portion sizes. Mindful eating, paired with the right ingredients and preparation methods, allows for a satisfying dessert experience without causing drastic fluctuations in blood sugar levels.

The Impact of Different Sweeteners on Blood Sugar Levels:

1. Natural Sweeteners: Natural sweeteners like stevia, erythritol, and monk fruit extract have little to no effect on blood sugar levels and are suitable alternatives for individuals with diabetes.

2. Artificial Sweeteners: Sugar substitutes like aspartame, sucralose, and saccharin have no impact on blood sugar and are commonly used in sugar-free desserts.

3. Sugar Alcohols: Sugar alcohols like xylitol, sorbitol, and mannitol have a minimal effect on blood sugar levels and are often used in low-carb desserts.

4. Sugar: Regular table sugar (sucrose) raises blood sugar levels and should be consumed in moderation by individuals with diabetes.

5. Natural Sugars: Naturally occurring sugars in fruits and dairy products, like fructose and lactose, should also be accounted for when planning desserts.

Diabetes-Friendly Dessert Recipes

1. Sugar-Free Chocolate Avocado Mousse: A rich and creamy mousse made with avocado, cocoa powder, and a natural sweetener like stevia.

2. Low-Carb Berry Crisp: A fruity dessert featuring mixed berries topped with a crumbly almond flour and coconut oil crust.

3. Almond Flour Cookies: Soft and chewy cookies made with almond flour, sugar-free sweetener, and a touch of cinnamon.

4. Greek Yogurt Parfait: Layers of Greek yogurt, fresh berries, and nuts, sweetened with a drizzle of honey or a low-carb sweetener.

5. Sugar-Free Lemon Bars: Tangy lemon bars made with almond flour crust and a sugar-free lemon filling.

6. Coconut Chia Pudding: A creamy chia seed pudding made with coconut milk and sweetened with a sugar substitute.

7. Baked Apples with Cinnamon: Sliced apples sprinkled with cinnamon and baked until tender, served with a dollop of sugar-free whipped cream.

8. Flourless Chocolate Cake: A decadent chocolate cake made with ground almonds or almond flour and sweetened with a natural sugar substitute.

9. Raspberry Coconut Popsicles: Refreshing popsicles made with coconut milk and fresh raspberries, sweetened with stevia.

10. Banana Nut Muffins: Moist and nutty muffins made with ripe bananas, almond flour, and chopped nuts.

11. No-Bake Cheesecake Bites: Mini cheesecake bites made with a nut crust and a creamy cheesecake filling sweetened with a sugar substitute.

12. Sugar-Free Pumpkin Pie: A classic pumpkin pie made with a low-carb crust and a pumpkin filling sweetened with a natural sugar substitute.

13. Chocolate Peanut Butter Protein Balls: Energy-boosting protein balls made with cocoa powder, peanut butter, and a low-carb sweetener.

14. Berry Frozen Yogurt: A guilt-free frozen treat made with Greek yogurt and mixed berries, sweetened with a natural sweetener.

15. Carrot Cake Cupcakes: Carrot cupcakes made with almond flour and grated carrots, topped with a cream cheese frosting sweetened with a sugar substitute.

Tips for Diabetes-Friendly Desserts

1. Portion Control: Enjoy desserts in moderation and be mindful of portion sizes to prevent excessive carbohydrate intake.

2. Balance with Protein and Fiber: Combining desserts with protein and fiber-rich ingredients can help stabilize blood sugar levels.

3. Use Low-Glycemic Ingredients: Choose ingredients with a low glycemic index to minimize their impact on blood sugar levels.

4. Monitor Blood Sugar Levels: Test blood sugar levels after trying new dessert recipes to understand their impact on individual blood sugar responses.

5. Enjoy Desserts with Meals: Consuming desserts as part of a balanced meal can help mitigate their effect on blood sugar levels.

6. Regular Exercise: Incorporating regular physical activity can improve blood sugar control and provide more flexibility in enjoying occasional desserts.

7. Consult with a Registered Dietitian: Working with a registered dietitian can help individuals with diabetes develop personalized dessert options that align with their dietary goals.

By embracing a mindful approach and exploring diabetes-friendly dessert recipes, individuals with diabetes can indulge in sweet treats while maintaining optimal blood sugar control.

It's essential to remember that no single dessert is suitable for everyone, and individual preferences and responses to sweeteners may vary.

Customizing recipes to suit personal tastes and dietary requirements is the key to crafting desserts that cater to individual health needs without compromising on flavor and satisfaction.

With the right knowledge and creativity, individuals with diabetes can experience the joy of desserts as part of a balanced and diabetes-friendly lifestyle.

Chapter Fourteen

Hydration and Kidney Health: The Vital Connection for Optimal Renal Function

Hydration plays a critical role in kidney health and overall well-being. The kidneys are essential organs responsible for filtering waste products, regulating fluid balance, and maintaining electrolyte levels in the body.

Proper hydration is crucial for supporting these functions and preventing kidney-related issues.

In this comprehensive guide, we will explore the importance of hydration for kidney health, the impact of dehydration on the kidneys, how to maintain optimal hydration levels, and practical tips for staying hydrated.

The Importance of Hydration for Kidney Health:
1. Waste Removal: Adequate hydration supports the kidneys' primary function of filtering waste

products from the blood and eliminating them through urine. When properly hydrated, the kidneys can efficiently remove waste, preventing the buildup of toxins in the body.

2. Electrolyte Balance: The kidneys help maintain the balance of essential electrolytes, such as sodium, potassium, and calcium. Proper hydration is crucial for supporting these electrolyte levels and preventing imbalances that can lead to health issues.

3. Blood Pressure Regulation: The kidneys play a key role in regulating blood pressure by adjusting the volume of blood and the amount of sodium excreted. Dehydration can lead to a decrease in blood volume, leading to increased blood pressure and putting additional strain on the kidneys.

4. Kidney Stone Prevention: Staying well-hydrated can reduce the risk of kidney stone formation. Sufficient water intake helps dilute urine, preventing the minerals and salts from crystallizing and forming stones.

5. Kidney Disease Prevention: Chronic dehydration is associated with an increased risk of developing kidney disease. Maintaining proper hydration levels may help reduce the risk of kidney damage and related complications.

The Impact of Dehydration on the Kidneys:
1. Decreased Filtration: Dehydration reduces blood flow to the kidneys, leading to decreased filtration efficiency. As a result, waste products and toxins may not be adequately eliminated, potentially causing kidney damage.

2. Concentrated Urine: When dehydrated, the kidneys produce more concentrated urine, which can contribute to the formation of kidney stones and urinary tract infections.

3. Reduced Blood Volume: Dehydration leads to a decrease in blood volume, causing the kidneys to conserve water and sodium. This response can result in elevated blood pressure and increased strain on the kidneys.

4. Electrolyte Imbalances: Insufficient hydration can lead to imbalances in essential electrolytes like sodium and potassium, which may negatively impact kidney function.

Maintaining Optimal Hydration Levels:

1. Drink Adequate Fluids: The general guideline for daily fluid intake is around 9-13 cups (2.2-3 liters) for women and 13-17 cups (3-4 liters) for men. Individual hydration requirements, however, could change depending on things like age, intensity of activity, and climate.

2. Listen to Thirst Cues: Thirst is the body's natural signal for water intake. Responding promptly to thirst cues is essential for maintaining hydration.

3. Monitor Urine Color: Urine color can be an indicator of hydration status. Light yellow or pale straw-colored urine generally indicates adequate hydration, while dark yellow or amber urine may signal dehydration.

4. Pay Attention to Sweat: In hot and humid conditions or during physical activity, increase fluid intake to compensate for water loss through sweat.

5. Include Water-Rich Foods: Fruits and vegetables with high water content, such as cucumbers, watermelon, oranges, and celery, can contribute to overall hydration.

6. Limit Dehydrating Beverages: Reduce or avoid beverages that can lead to dehydration, such as caffeinated and alcoholic drinks.

Practical Tips for Staying Hydrated:
1. Carry a Water Bottle: Keep a reusable water bottle with you throughout the day to encourage regular sips and easy access to hydration.

2. Set Hydration Goals: Set daily hydration goals and track your fluid intake to ensure you are meeting your hydration needs.

3. Create Hydration Reminders: Set alarms or use smartphone apps to remind yourself to drink water regularly.

4. Infuse Water: Add natural flavors to water by infusing it with fresh fruits, herbs, or cucumbers to make it more enjoyable.

5. Drink Before Meals: Drink a glass of water before meals to boost hydration and potentially help with appetite control.

6. Hydrate During and After Exercise: Drink water before, during, and after physical activity to stay hydrated and replace fluid loss.

7. Monitor Hydration during Illness: During illnesses that cause vomiting, diarrhea, or fever, pay extra attention to hydration and replace lost fluids.

Hydration and Kidney Health: Frequently Asked Questions

1. How does dehydration affect kidney function?

Dehydration reduces blood flow to the kidneys, leading to decreased filtration efficiency. This can result in the accumulation of waste products and toxins in the body, potentially causing kidney damage. Dehydration also contributes to the formation of kidney stones and urinary tract infections.

2. How much water should I drink daily for kidney health?

The general guideline for daily fluid intake is around 9-13 cups (2.2-3 liters) for women and 13-17 cups (3-4 liters) for men. Individual hydration requirements, however, could change depending on things like age, intensity of activity, and climate.

3. Can staying well-hydrated prevent kidney stones?

Yes, staying well-hydrated can help prevent kidney stone formation. Sufficient water intake helps dilute urine, preventing the minerals and salts from crystallizing and forming stones.

4. Are there any beverages I should avoid to maintain kidney health?

It's best to limit or avoid beverages that can lead to dehydration, such as caffeinated and alcoholic drinks. These beverages can have diuretic effects, leading to increased water loss through urine.

5. Can dehydration contribute to kidney disease?

Chronic dehydration is associated with an increased risk of developing kidney disease. Proper hydration is essential for supporting kidney function and reducing the risk of kidney damage and related complications.

In Summary

Maintaining proper hydration is essential for kidney health and overall well-being. Adequate fluid intake supports the kidneys' vital functions, including waste removal, electrolyte balance, and blood pressure regulation.

Staying hydrated can prevent dehydration-related complications, such as kidney stones and urinary tract infections, and reduce the risk of kidney damage. By listening to thirst cues, monitoring urine color, and incorporating water-rich foods, individuals can support optimal kidney function and promote overall health through proper hydration.

It is crucial to consult with healthcare providers or registered dietitians to ensure that individual hydration needs are met, especially for individuals with specific medical conditions or kidney health concerns.

With a mindful approach to hydration, individuals can safeguard their kidney health and enjoy the numerous benefits of being well-hydrated.

Chapter Fifteen

Planning Meals for Long-Term Health: A Holistic Approach to Nourishment

Meal planning is a key component of long-term health and well-being. It involves deliberate and thoughtful choices about the foods we consume to support our nutritional needs, maintain a healthy weight, and prevent chronic diseases.

A well-rounded meal plan considers various aspects, including balanced nutrition, portion control, dietary preferences, and individual health goals. In this comprehensive guide, we will explore the benefits of meal planning for long-term health, the principles of balanced nutrition, strategies for meal preparation, and practical tips to create sustainable and nutritious meal plans.

The Benefits of Meal Planning for Long-Term Health

1. Nutritional Adequacy: Meal planning ensures that meals are nutritionally balanced and provide the necessary nutrients the body needs for optimal functioning. A well-planned diet can contribute to overall health, energy levels, and disease prevention.

2. Portion Control: Planning meals in advance helps control portion sizes, preventing overeating and promoting weight management.

3. Time and Money Savings: Meal planning can save time and money by reducing food waste and unnecessary trips to the grocery store. It also allows for bulk cooking and utilizing ingredients efficiently.

4. Dietary Variety: A well-thought-out meal plan encourages dietary diversity, exposing the body to a wide range of nutrients and promoting a healthier gut microbiome.

5. Stress Reduction: Knowing what to eat and having meals prepared in advance can reduce stress and decision fatigue related to daily meal choices.

6. Weight Management: Meal planning supports weight management goals by promoting portion control and balanced nutrition, helping individuals achieve and maintain a healthy weight.

Principles of Balanced Nutrition in Meal Planning:

1. Macronutrients: A balanced meal should include adequate portions of carbohydrates, proteins, and fats. Carbohydrates provide energy, proteins support tissue repair and growth, and fats play essential roles in nutrient absorption and hormone regulation.

2. Micronutrients: Ensure meals contain a variety of vitamins and minerals from fruits, vegetables, whole grains, nuts, and seeds. These micronutrients support various physiological functions and help prevent nutrient deficiencies.

3. Fiber: Incorporate fiber-rich foods like whole grains, fruits, vegetables, and legumes to support digestive health and maintain steady blood sugar levels.

4. Hydration: Include sufficient water and fluids throughout the day to stay hydrated and support kidney and overall health.

5. Mindful Eating: Encourage mindful eating practices, such as eating slowly, savoring flavors, and paying attention to hunger and fullness cues.

Strategies for Meal Preparation and Planning:

1. Weekly Menu Planning: Plan meals for the week ahead, considering family preferences, dietary goals, and seasonal availability of ingredients.

2. Batch Cooking: Prepare large batches of staple foods like grains, beans, and proteins to use as building blocks for various meals throughout the week.

3. Use Leftovers Wisely: Repurpose leftovers into new dishes to reduce food waste and save time in the kitchen.

4. Prepare Snacks: Plan and prepare healthy snacks to have on hand for moments of hunger or cravings.

5. Cook in Bulk: Cook multiple portions of soups, stews, and casseroles to freeze and enjoy on busy days.

6. Smart Grocery Shopping: Make a shopping list based on the weekly meal plan to ensure you have all the necessary ingredients on hand.

7. Portion Control: Practice portion control by using smaller plates and containers to avoid overeating.

8. Plan for Variety: Aim to include a wide range of colors, flavors, and textures in your meals to make them more enjoyable and nutritious.

9. Seasonal Eating: Incorporate seasonal produce into your meal plan to benefit from fresher and more flavorful ingredients.

1. Consider Dietary Preferences: Take into account personal dietary preferences and cultural influences to create a meal plan that aligns with individual tastes and lifestyle.

2. Set Realistic Goals: Establish achievable dietary goals that contribute to overall health and well-being. Avoid extreme diets or restrictions that may not be sustainable in the long term.

3. Plan Balanced Meals: Ensure each meal includes a variety of food groups, such as lean proteins, whole grains, healthy fats, and plenty of fruits and vegetables.

4. Gradual Changes: Make dietary changes gradually to allow for better adaptation and long-term adherence.

5. Seek Professional Guidance: Consult with a registered dietitian or healthcare provider for personalized advice and support in creating a meal plan that meets specific health needs and goals.

6. Mindful Indulgences: Allow for occasional indulgences or treats while keeping overall nutrition in mind. Maintaining good eating patterns requires balance.

7. Include Physical Activity: Pair meal planning with regular physical activity to optimize long-term health and well-being.

In conclusion, meal planning is a powerful tool for supporting long-term health and well-being. A well-thought-out meal plan ensures balanced nutrition, portion control, and dietary variety, contributing to overall health, weight management, and disease prevention. By incorporating strategies like weekly menu planning, batch cooking, and mindful eating practices, individuals can create sustainable and nutritious meal plans that align with their dietary preferences and health goals.

Consultation with a registered dietitian or healthcare professional can provide personalized guidance and support in developing meal plans that cater to individual needs and contribute to long-term health and well-being.

With a mindful and holistic approach to meal planning, individuals can enjoy nourishing and satisfying meals that promote optimal health and enhance their quality of life.

Conclusion

"Deliciously Diabetic: A Nourishing Renal Diet Cookbook for Healthy Kidneys" is a comprehensive and invaluable resource for individuals with diabetes and kidney health concerns.

This cookbook offers a wide array of delicious and nutrient-rich recipes that cater to both diabetic and renal dietary requirements. By focusing on the principles of balanced nutrition, portion control, and mindful eating, this cookbook provides practical solutions for managing blood sugar levels and supporting optimal kidney function.

Understanding the intricate link between diabetes and kidney disease is crucial, and this cookbook's introductory chapters offer valuable insights into these health conditions. Readers gain a deeper understanding of diabetic nephropathy, risk factors for diabetic kidney disease, mechanisms of kidney damage in diabetes, and diagnostic and preventive strategies.

The cookbook also emphasizes the importance of lifestyle modifications, medications, and nutritional considerations that can significantly impact diabetes and kidney health.

With the cookbook's 15 thoughtfully crafted chapters, readers embark on a culinary journey that covers an extensive range of topics. From "Navigating a Diabetic Renal Diet" to "Understanding Blood Glucose Control" and "Hydration and Kidney Health," this cookbook addresses all aspects of diabetes and kidney health with precision and care.

The collection of delectable and kidney-friendly recipes encourages readers to relish their meals while promoting overall health and well-being.

From wholesome breakfast delights to satisfying lunches, creative snacks, and delightful dinners, this cookbook effortlessly blends taste and health in every dish. The incorporation of nutrient-rich ingredients, mindful portion control, and a diverse array of cuisines ensures that individuals with diabetes and renal concerns can enjoy a flavorful and nourishing dining experience.

As readers embark on their journey to better health with the aid of this cookbook, they are encouraged to collaborate with healthcare providers and dietitians for personalized guidance and support.

By adhering to the principles and recipes outlined in "Deliciously Diabetic: A Nourishing Renal Diet Cookbook for Healthy Kidneys," individuals can confidently embrace a balanced, flavorful, and kidney-friendly diet to thrive in their pursuit of long-term health and well-being.